T0233754

SpringerBriefs in Child Health

Series editor
Angelo P. Giardino

More information about this series at http://www.springer.com/series/10138

Rashmi Shetgiri • Dorothy L. Espelage
Leslie Carroll

Practical Strategies
for Clinical Management
of Bullying

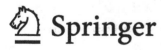
Springer

Rashmi Shetgiri
Los Angeles Biomedical Research Institute
   at Harbor-UCLA Medical Center
Torrance, CA, USA

Dorothy L. Espelage
University of Illinois at Urbana-Champaign
Champaign, IL, USA

Leslie Carroll
Family Voices
Albuquerque, NM, USA

ISSN 2192-3698
SpringerBriefs in Child Health
ISBN 978-3-319-15475-6
DOI 10.1007/978-3-319-15476-3

ISSN 2192-3701   (electronic)

ISBN 978-3-319-15476-3   (eBook)

Library of Congress Control Number: 2015932503

Springer Cham Heidelberg New York Dordrecht London

Printed on acid-free paper

Springer International Publishing AG Switzerland is part of Springer Science+Business Media (www.springer.com)

Contents

Chapter 1
Introduction

Bullying is a significant problem for children and adolescents. One out of three children in the United States is involved in bullying. It is highly likely, therefore, that parents, clinicians, and members of child-serving organizations are likely to encounter children who have been bullied, who have bullied others, or both. Recent media reports have drawn a great deal of attention to the negative outcomes associated with bullying, including several high-profile instances of "bullycide." There has not, however, been much clarity about how to identify and effectively intervene with bullying. Given the high rates of child involvement in bullying, it is important for parents and other adults to know how to respond effectively. Clinicians can play an important role in educating parents and communities about this issue. The chapters in this book focus on the current research on bullying, including bullying trends and consequences; school and community-based interventions; current and emerging policy and advocacy regarding bullying; and identifying and intervening in bullying in the clinical setting. The book brings together research, policy, and practical strategies to arm parents, clinicians, and communities with the knowledge to successfully intervene in child bullying.

© Springer International Publishing Switzerland 2015
R. Shetgiri et al., *Practical Strategies for Clinical Management of Bullying*,
SpringerBriefs in Child Health, DOI 10.1007/978-3-319-15476-3_1

Chapter 2
Bullying Trends, Correlates, Consequences, and Characteristics

Bullying is regarded as a significant problem in the US among school-aged youth. Rates for bullying among school-age youth range from 10 % to 30 % internationally with a notable increase during the middle school years (Cook et al. 2010; Espelage et al. in press). More specifically, in the US, between 15 % and 23 % of elementary students and 20–28 % of secondary school students report being bullied within a 6-month to 1-year period (Carlyle and Steinman 2007; National Center for Educational Statistics 2011; Turner et al. 2011). Also, approximately nine to eleven percent of youth report being called hate-related words having to do with their race, religion, ethnic background, and/or sexual orientation (Robers et al. 2013).

Rates appear to vary across sex and race/ethnicity. Many studies report that boys are more likely to engage in physical bullying than girls (Espelage et al. 2014; Nansel et al. 2001; Varjas et al. 2009). During the 1990s, much research supported the notion that girls are socialized to exercise more relational forms of aggression or social bullying, whereas boys engage in multiple forms of aggression (Neal 2007). Despite these findings, several studies have failed to document significant sex differences in relational aggression or social forms of bullying (Card et al. 2008; Crick et al. 1997). In addition to sex, race/ethnicity has been another major focus of research, and higher frequency of bullying perpetration and victimization among African-American students has been reported (Belgrave 2009; Koo et al. 2012; Wang et al. 2009). When African-American youth report more bullying perpetration (Carlyle and Steinman 2007; Espelage et al. 2012; Low and Espelage 2012), these studies have yielded small effect sizes. Thus, the research on both sex and race/ethnicity differences in reports of bullying perpetration are inconsistent and limited.

© Springer International Publishing Switzerland 2015
R. Shetgiri et al., *Practical Strategies for Clinical Management of Bullying*,
SpringerBriefs in Child Health, DOI 10.1007/978-3-319-15476-3_2

Definitional Issues

Prevalence rates vary in large part because of differences in how bullying is defined and measured (AERA 2013; Rodkin et al. in press). One of the first predominant definitions of bullying that continues to be used in the literature and in the legal arena is as follows: "A student is being bullied or victimized when he or she is exposed, repeatedly and over time, to negative actions on the part of one or more students." (Olweus 2010, p. 11). More recent definitions of bullying emphasize observable or non-observable aggressive behaviors, the repetitive nature of these behaviors, and the imbalance of power between the individual/group perpetrator and victim (Gladden et al. 2014; Ybarra et al. 2014). An imbalance of power exists when the perpetrator or group of perpetrators have more physical, social, or intellectual power than the victim. In a recent examination of a nationally-representative study, early and late adolescents that perceived their perpetrator as having more power reported greater adverse outcomes (e.g., depression, suicidal ideation) than victims who did not perceive a power differential (Ybarra et al. 2014).

For the last 3 years, the Department of Education and the Centers for Disease Control and Prevention have worked closely to develop a uniform *research* definition. This group defined bullying as follows: "Bullying is any unwanted aggressive behavior(s) by another youth or group of youths who are not siblings or current dating partners that involves an observed or perceived power imbalance and is repeated multiple times or is highly likely to be repeated. Bullying may inflict harm or distress on the targeted youth including physical, psychological, social, or educational harm." (Gladden et al. 2014). These behaviors include verbal and physical aggression that ranges in severity from making threats, spreading rumors, and social exclusion, to physical attacks causing injury. Bullying can occur face-to-face and/or through technology (e.g., cell phones, computers).

Correlates and Consequences of Bully Perpetration and Victimization

Academic Outcomes Several national and international research studies relying on cross-sectional data have documented that experiences of being victimized or bullying other students are associated with decreased academic achievement. For example, findings from a sample of 7th, 9th, and 11th graders in an urban public school district, revealed that for each 1-point increase in grade point average, the odds of being a victim versus a bystander decreased by 10 % (Glew et al. 2008). These associations also are found when students are followed over time in longitudinal studies (e.g., Juvonen et al. 2011; Schwartz et al. 2005). Juvonen and colleagues (2011) documented that peer victimization can account for an average 1.5 letter grade decrease in one academic subject (e.g., math) across 3 years of middle school.

Moreover, the researchers found that greater self-reported victimization was associated with lower grades and lower teacher-rated academic engagement. However, a meta-analytic review of 33 cross-sectional studies conducted by Nakamoto and Schwartz (2010) reported that empirical research on this association has produced an incongruent pattern of findings and modest correlations. In fact, these authors reported a small but significant negative correlation between peer victimization and academic achievement. Friendship quality and peer social support appear to have a complex moderating role in the association between peer victimization and academic performance (Schwartz et al. 2008).

Psychiatric Disorders, Depression, and Suicidality Few studies directly assess the relationship between bullying and mental health disorders (Copeland et al. 2013; Fanti and Kimonis 2013; Kumpulainen et al. 2001). Kumpulainen et al. (2001), using an epidemiological sample of second graders from Finland, found that children who were classified as bullies (children who bully others but are not bullied themselves) and bully-victims (children who both bully and are bullied) had high rates of psychiatric disorders relative to uninvolved children, largely for externalizing behaviors like attention deficit/hyperactivity disorder, oppositional defiant disorder, and conduct disorder. In particular, bully-victims were likely to have more severe problems and to have used mental health services. Similar findings emerge in Copeland et al.'s (2013) U.S. Great Smoky Mountain study; children and youth who self-reported involvement in bullying were more likely than uninvolved youth to be diagnosed via child- and parent-reports with disruptive and substance use disorders; bully-victims were additionally at risk for internalizing disorders including depression and suicidality. These youth were later assessed for psychiatric disorders such as depression, suicidality, anxiety, panic disorder, agoraphobia, antisocial personality disorder, and alcohol and marijuana abuse between the ages of 19 and 26 (Copeland et al. 2013). Youth who bullied during childhood were no different than children not involved in bullying on any of the nine long-term outcomes examined for except antisocial personality disorder. Childhood victims of bullying had higher rates of depression, anxiety, panic disorder, and agoraphobia as young adults. Bully-victims had the highest rates of depression, suicidality, anxiety, and panic disorder of all the groups. Other studies support these findings indicating that victims of bullying report significant psychosomatic problems and report depression later in life (Ttofi et al. 2011).

The majority of extant research indicates that involvement in bullying in any capacity is associated with higher rates of suicidal ideation and behaviors (Kim and Leventhal 2008). Most of the research on the links between bully/peer victimization and suicidal behaviors has been conducted outside of the US, but a 2009 paper examined the association between peer victimization and suicidal ideation and attempts across three nationally-representative samples of US adolescents (Kaminski and Fang 2009). Youth victimized by their peers were 2.4 times more likely to report suicidal ideation and 3.3 times more likely to report a suicide attempt than youth who reported not being bullied.

Although there is fairly consistent evidence that there is increased suicide risk for those involved in bullying, evidence suggests that risk might vary for youth who are bullies, victims, and bully-victims. For instance, some studies have shown that the association between suicidal ideation and bullying is stronger for targets of bullying than for perpetrators (e.g., Rigby and Slee 1999). Another study, however, found that after controlling for depression, the association between bullying and suicidal ideation was strongest for bully perpetrators (Kaltiala-Heino et al. 1999). Another study of middle school youth reported that the bully-suicide association was minimized when depression and delinquency were considered for all youth (Espelage and Holt 2013). Whereas multiple studies have found that bully-victims report more suicidal ideation and behaviors than uninvolved youth, victims, or perpetrators (e.g., Klomek et al. 2007), there are other studies that do not support this pattern. For instance, Herba and colleagues (2008) found that there were no differences in levels of suicidal ideation between bully-victims and uninvolved youth. These studies point to the complexity of assessing suicide risk based on the level of involvement youth play in the bully-victim dynamic.

Similarly, mixed findings exist with regard to whether the association between bullying and suicidal ideation varies by sex. One study found that victimization from bullying increases the likelihood of suicidal ideation among boys 2.5 times, and almost 4 times among girls (Hinduja and Patchin 2010). Klomek and colleagues (2009) found that bullying victimization at age 8 was associated with later suicide attempts and completed suicides after controlling for depression and conduct problems, but this was the case only for girls. Among boys, the relationship between victimization and suicidal ideation was mediated by depression and conduct disorder. The authors speculate that this sex difference might have emerged given that girls are more likely to experience relational victimization (e.g., indirect, manipulative, social or emotion-based) whereas boys are more likely to experience physical victimization (physical aggression, fights), and relational victimization might have a more long-lasting impact. On the other hand, other studies have found that boys might be at greater risk. For instance, male bullies showed higher than average levels of suicidal ideation in one study of a community population (Rigby and Slee 1999), and in a sample of Italian youth seeking psychological help suicidal ideation was predicted by being bullied at school only for boys (Laukkanen et al. 2005). Overall, research comparing sexual and gender minority and heterosexual youth has consistently shown that sexual minority youth report higher levels of suicidality (Eisenberg and Resnick 2006; Remafedi et al. 1998; Robinson and Espelage 2011; Russell and Toomey 2012). The existing research on the relationship between bullying involvement and suicide suggests that bullying may be a contributor to suicidality, however, other factors also may contribute to this relationship.

Delinquency, Criminal Activity, and Alcohol/Drug Use Only recently, have studies examined the link between bullying involvement and later delinquency and/or criminal behavior. In a 2011 meta-analysis, bullying perpetration at age 14 led to higher violent conviction rates between ages 15–20, lower job status at age 18, increased drug use from ages 27–32, and relationship problems by age 48

(Farrington and Ttofi 2011). Further, Hemphill and colleagues (2011) found that greater bullying perpetration among Australian youth in Year 7 of school was associated with a two-fold increase in binge drinking and marijuana use when these students were in Year 10 of school. From the US-based Raising Healthy Children project, childhood bullying in grade 5 was associated with heavy drinking and marijuana use at age 21 (Kim et al. 2011). Other studies have shown longitudinal associations between bullying among older adolescents and associations with heavy drinking and marijuana use into adulthood, but these studies often do not examine the potential mediating effects of family influence on the relationship between bullying and substance use.

Characteristics of Bullies and Victims

Children who bully are often believed to be insecure, aggressive, and lacking empathy. Although this is true for some bullies (Smokowski and Kopasz 2005), all bullies do not fit this profile. Some bullies have high self-esteem, good social skills, and are considered popular among their peers; they may use bullying as a strategy to attain social dominance (Smokowski and Kopasz 2005; Barker et al. 2008; Juvonen et al. 2003). Other children who bully may be involved in high-risk behaviors such as drug use, demonstrate behavioral problems such as defiance, attention deficit disorder, or conduct disorder, and may be less engaged in school (Smokowski and Kopasz 2005; Juvonen et al. 2003). It also is important to recognize that most children who bully do so for a short period of time. Children who bully others during middle school often cease to do so by the end of high school, with almost 90 % of children discontinuing involvement in bullying over time (Pepler et al. 2008).

Risk factors for child engagement in bullying perpetration include poor parent-child involvement and communication, use of corporal punishment in the home, family conflict, and exposure to violence in the home in the form of child abuse/neglect or domestic violence (Espelage et al. 2000; Yang et al. 2006; Spriggs et al. 2001; Bowes et al. 2009). Parental mental health also may influence child socioemotional development and involvement in bullying (Georgiou 2008; Kane and Garber 2004; Ramchandani et al. 2005). This relationship may be mediated by an influence on parenting behaviors (Georgiou 2008; McLearn et al. 2006). Paternal involvement in bullying in childhood is associated with child bullying, with children of fathers who bullied others in childhood having a higher likelihood of bullying others as well (Farrington 1993).

Children who are victimized by bullying also are a heterogeneous group. Passive victims are characterized as those who are less assertive, more sensitive, anxious, or insecure than their peers, or may be physically smaller or weaker than others (Smokowski and Kopasz 2005; Pellegrini et al. 1999). They also may have difficulty making friends with other children in their peer group (Smokowski and Kopasz 2005; Pellegrini et al. 1999). Proactive or aggressive victims are those who are victimized by others and respond with aggression, sometimes by bullying others (Smokowski and Kopasz 2005). Bully-victims may include this group, as well as those who transition from bullying to victimization, or from victimization to bullying, over time. Bully-victims are at the highest risk of negative outcomes of any of the groups of children involved in bullying. They are more socially-isolated than their peers, have higher rates of internalizing and externalizing disorders, and are least well-liked by peers and adults (Smokowski and Kopasz 2005; Barker et al. 2008).

References

American Educational Research Association. (2013). *Prevention of bullying in schools, colleges, and universities: research report and recommendations*. Washington, DC: American Educational Research Association.

Barker, E. D., Arsenault, L., Brendgen, M., et al. (2008). Joint development of bullying and victimization in adolescence: relations to delinquency and self-harm. *Journal of the American Academy of Child and Adolescent Psychiatry, 47*(9), 1030–1038.

Belgrave, F. Z. (2009). *African-American girls: reframing perceptions and changing experiences*. New York: Springer.

Bowes, L., Arseneault, L., Maughan, B., et al. (2009). School, neighborhood, and family factors are associated with children's bullying involvement: a nationally representative longitudinal study. *Journal of the American Academy of Child and Adolescent Psychiatry, 48*(5), 545–553.

Card, N., Stuckey, B., Sawalani, G., & Little, T. (2008). Direct and indirect aggression during childhood and adolescence: a meta-analytic review of gender differences, intercorrelations, and relations to maladjustment. *Child Development, 79*, 1185–1229.

Carlyle, K. E., & Steinman, K. J. (2007). Demographic differences in the prevalence, co-occurrence, and correlates of adolescent bullying at school. *Journal of School Health, 9*, 623–629. doi:10.1111/j.1746-1561.2007.00242.x.

Cook, C. R., Williams, K. R., Guerra, N. G., Kim, T. E., & Sadek, S. (2010). Predictors of bullying and victimization in childhood and adolescence: a meta-analytic investigation. *School Psychology Quarterly, 25*, 65–83.

Copeland, W. E., Wolke, D., Angold, A., & Costello, E. J. (2013). Adult psychiatric outcomes of bullying and being bullies by peers in childhood and adolescence. *JAMA Psychiatry, 70*, 419–426.

Crick, N. R., Casas, J. F., & Mosher, M. (1997). Relational and overt aggression in preschool. *Developmental Psychology, 33*, 579–588.

Eisenberg, M. E., & Resnick, M. D. (2006). Suicidality among gay, lesbian and bisexual youth: the role of protective factors. *Journal of Adolescent Health, 39*, 662–668. doi:10.1016/j.jadohealth.2006.04.024.

Espelage, D. L., & Holt, M. (2013). Suicidal ideation & school bullying experiences after controlling for depression & delinquency. *Journal of Adolescent Health, 53*, S27–S31.

Espelage, D. L., Bosworth, K., & Simon, T. R. (2000). Examining the social context of bullying behaviors in early adolescence. *Journal of Counseling and Development, 78*(3), 326–333.

Espelage, D.L., Basile, K.C., & Hamburger, M.E. (2012). Bullying experiences and co-occurring sexual violence perpetration among middle school students: shared and unique risk factors. *Journal of Adolescent Health, 50*, 60–65.

Espelage, D. L., Low, S., Rao, M. A., Hong, J. S., & Little, T. (2014). Family violence, bullying, fighting, and substance use among adolescents: a longitudinal transactional model. *Journal of Research on Adolescence, 24*(2), 337–349.

Espelage, D. L., Hong, J. S., Rao, M., & Thornber, R. (in press). Social-ecological factors associated with bullying perpetration among early adolescents across the elementary-middle school transition. *Violence & Victims*.

Fanti, K. A., & Kimonis, E. R. (2013). Bullying and victimization: the role of conduct problems and psychopathic traits. *Journal of Research on Adolescence, 22*, 617–631.

Farrington, D. P. (1993). Understanding and preventing bullying. In M. Tonry (Ed.), *Crime and justice: a review of research* (pp. 381–458). Chicago: University of Chicago Press.

Farrington, D. P., & Ttofi, M. M. (2011). Bullying as a predictor of offending, violence and later life outcomes. *Criminal Behaviour and Mental Health, 21*(2), 90–98. doi:http://dx.doi.org/10.1002/cbm.801.

Georgiou, S. N. (2008). Bullying and victimization at school: the role of mothers. *British Journal of Educational Psychology, 78*, 109–125.

Gladden, R. M., Vivolo-Kantor, A. M., Hamburger, M. E., & Lumpkin, C. D. (2014). *Bullying surveillance among youths: uniform definitions for public health and recommended data elements, version 1.0*. Atlanta: National Center for Injury Prevention and Control, Centers for Disease Control and Prevention and U.S. Department of Education.

Glew, G. M., Fan, M. Y., Katon, W., & Rivara, F. P. (2008). Bullying and school safety. *The Journal of Pediatrics, 152*, 123–128.

Hemphill, F. C., & Vanneman, A. (2011). *Achievement gaps: how Hispanic and white students in public schools perform in mathematics and reading on the national assessment of educational progress*. Statistical Analysis Report. NCES 2011–459. Institute of Education Sciences, U.S. Department of Education. Washington; DC

Herba, C. M., Ferdinand, R. F., Stijnen, T., Veenstra, R., Oldehinkel, A. J., Ormel, J., et al. (2008). Victimisation and suicide ideation in the TRAILS study: specific vulnerabilities of victims. *Journal of Child Psychiatry & Psychology, 49*, 867–876.

Hinduja, S., & Patchin, J. W. (2010). Bullying, cyberbullying, and suicide. *Archives of Suicide Research, 14*, 206–221.

Juvonen, J., Graham, S., & Schuster, M. A. (2003). Bullying among young adolescents: the strong, the weak, and the troubled. *Pediatrics, 112*(6), 1231–1237.

Juvonen, J., Wang, Y., & Espinoza, G. (2011). Bullying experiences and compromised academic performance across middle school grades. *Journal of Early Adolescence, 31*, 152–173.

Kaltiala-Heino, R., Rimpela, M., Marttunen, M., Rimpela, A., & Rantanen, P. (1999). Bullying, depression, and suicidal ideation in Finnish adolescents. *British Medical Journal, 319*, 348–351.

Kaminski, J. W., & Fang, X. (2009). Victimization by peers and adolescent suicide in three US samples. *Journal of Pediatrics, 155*, 638–688.

Kane, P., & Garber, J. (2004). The relations among depression in fathers, children's psychopathology, and father-child conflict: a meta-analysis. *Clinical Psychology Review, 24*, 339–360.

Kim, Y. S., & Leventhal, B. (2008). Bullying and suicide. A review. *International Journal of Adolescent Medicine and Health, 20*(2), 133–154.

Kim, M. J., Catalano, R. F., Haggerty, K. P., & Abbott, R. D. (2011). Bullying at elementary school and problem behaviour in young adulthood: a study of bullying, violence and substance use from age 11 to age 21. *Criminal Behaviour and Mental Health, 21*(2), 136–144.

Klomek, A., Marrocco, F., Kleinman, M., Schonfeld, I. S., & Gould, M. S. (2007). Bullying, depression, and suicidality in adolescents. *Journal of American Academic of Child & Adolescent Psychology, 46*, 40–49.

Klomek, A. B., Sourander, A., Niemela, S., Kumpulainen, K., Piha, J., Tamminen, T., et al. (2009). Childhood bullying behaviors as a risk for suicide attempts and completed suicides: a population-based birth cohort study. *Journal of American Academy of Child & Adolescence Psychology, 48*, 254–261.

Koo, D. J., Peguero, A. A., & Shekarkhar, Z. (2012). Gender, immigration, and school victimization. *Victims & Offenders, 7*, 77–96. doi:10.1080/15564886.2011.629773.

Kumpulainen, K., Räsänen, E., & Puura, K. (2001). Psychiatric disorders and the use of mental health services among children involved in bullying. *Aggressive Behavior, 27*(2), 102–110.

Laukkanen, E., Honkalampi, K., Hintikka, J., Hintikka, U., & Lehtonen, J. (2005). Suicidal ideation among help-seeking adolescents. *Archives of Suicide Research, 9*, 45–55.

Low, S., & Espelage, D. L. (2012). Differentiating cyber bullying perpetration from other forms of peer aggression: commonalities across race, individual, and family predictors. *Psychology of Violence, 3*, 39–52.

McLearn, K. T., Minkovitz, C. S., Strobino, D. M., et al. (2006). The timing of maternal depressive symptoms and mothers' parenting practices with young children: implications for pediatric practice. *Pediatrics, 118*, e174–e182.

Nakamoto, J., & Schwartz, D. (2010). Is peer victimization associated with academic achievement? a meta-analytic review. *Social Development, 19*, 221–242.

Nansel, T. R., Overpeck, M., Pilla, R. S., Ruan, W., Simons-Morton, B., & Scheidt, P. (2001). Bullying behaviors among US youth: prevalence and association with psychosocial adjustment. *Journal of the American Medical Association, 285*, 2094–2100.

National Center for Education Statistics (2011). Achievement Gaps: How Hispanic and White Students in Public Schools Perform in Mathematics and Reading on the National Assessment of Educational Progress. *Statistical Analysis Report. NCES* 2011–459.

Neal, J. W. (2007). Why social networks matter: a structural approach to the study of relational forms of aggression in middle childhood and adolescence. *Child and Youth Care Forum, 36*, 195–211.

Olweus, D. (2010). Understanding and researching bullying: some critical issues. In S. R. Jimerson, S. M. Swearer, & D. L. Espelage (Eds.), *Handbook of bullying in schools: an international perspective* (pp. 9–34). New York: Routledge.

Pellegrini, A. D., Bartini, M., & Brooks, F. (1999). School bullies, victims, and aggressive victims: factors relating to group affiliation and victimization in early adolescence. *Journal of Educational Psychology, 91*(2), 216–224.

Pepler, D., Jiang, D., Craig, W., et al. (2008). Developmental trajectories of bullying and associated factors. *Child Development, 79*(2), 325–338.

Ramchandani, P., Stein, A., Evans, J., et al. (2005). Paternal depression in the postnatal period and child development: a prospective population study. *Lancet, 365*, 2201–2205.

Remafedi, G., French, S., Story, M., Resnick, M. D., & Blum, R. (1998). The relationship between suicide risk and sexual orientation: results of a population-based study. *American Journal of Public Health, 88*, 57–60.

Rigby, K., & Slee, P. (1999). Suicidal ideation among adolescent school children, involvement in bully-victim problems and perceived social support. *Suicide and Life-Threatening Behavior, 29*, 119–130.

Robers, S., Kemp, J., & Truman, J. (2013). *Indicators of school crime and safety: 2012*. NCES 2013-036/NCJ 241446. Washington, DC: National Center for Education Statistics.

Robinson, J. P., & Espelage, D. L. (2011). Inequities in educational and psychological outcomes between LGBTQ and straight students in middle and high school. *Educational Researcher, 40*, 315–330.

Rodkin, P. C., Espelage, D. L., & Hanish, L. D. (in press). A relational perspective on the social ecology of bullying. *American Psychologist*.

Russell, S. T., & Toomey, R. B. (2012). Men's sexual orientation and suicide: evidence for U.S. adolescent-specific risk. *Social Science and Medicine, 74*, 523–529. doi:10.1016/j.socscimed.2010.07.038.

Schwartz, D., Gorman, A. H., Nakamoto, J., & Toblin, R. (2005). Victimization in the peer group and children's academic functioning. *Journal of Educational Psychology, 97*, 425–435.

Schwartz, D., Gorman, A. H., Dodge, K. A., Pettit, G. S., & Bates, J. E. (2008). Friendships with peers who are low or high in aggression as moderators of the link between peer victimization and declines in academic functioning. *Journal of Abnormal Child Psychology, 36*, 719–730.

Smokowski, P. R., & Kopasz, K. H. (2005). Bullying in school: an overview of types, effects, family characteristics, and intervention strategies. *Children and Schools, 37*(2), 101–110.

Spriggs, A. L., Iannotti, R. J., Nansel, T. R., et al. (2001). Adolescent bullying involvement and perceived family, peer, and school relations: commonalities and differences across race/ethnicity. *Journal of Adolescent Health, 41*, 283–293.

Ttofi, M. M., Farrington, D. P., Lösel, F., Loeber, R. (2011). Do the victims of school bullies tend to become depressed later in life? A systematic review and meta analysis of longitudinal studies. *Journal of Aggression, Conflict and Peace Research, 3*(2), 63–73.

Turner, H. A., Finkelhor, D., Hamby, S. L., Shattuck, A., & Ormrod, R. K. (2011). Specifying type and location of peer victimization in a national sample of children and youth. *Journal of Youth and Adolescence, 40*(8), 1052–1067.

Varjas, K., Henrich, C. C., & Meyers, J. (2009). Urban middle school students' perceptions of bullying, cyberbullying, and school safety. *Journal of School Violence, 8,* 159–176. doi:10.1080/15388220802074165.

Wang, J., Iannotti, R. J., & Nansel, T. R. (2009). School bullying among adolescents in the United States: Physical, verbal, relational, and cyber. *Journal of Adolescent health, 45*(4), 368–375.

Yang, S., Kim, J., Kim, S., et al. (2006). Bullying and victimization behaviors in boys and girls at South Korean primary schools. *Journal of the American Academy of Child and Adolescent Psychiatry, 45,* 69–77.

Ybarra, M., Espelage, D. L., & Mitchell, K. J. (2014). Differentiating youth who are bullied from other victims of peer-aggression: the importance of differential power and repetition. *Journal of Adolescent Health. 55*(2), 293–300.

Chapter 3
"Sometimes People Mean?": A Parent's Perspective on Victimization of Children with Special Health Care Needs

Bullying among children with special health care needs is a highly-charged topic for parents, and writing about it brings not only opportunities to examine the research, but also some unexpected feelings. Reading articles, blogs, and watching YouTube videos of parents working together with teachers, administrators, and legislators to prevent bullying is inspiring; it is through these collaborative efforts that bullying prevention will succeed. But my own child's story keeps creeping in; unresolved outcomes from bullying experiences in the past, which may never be completely resolved. The experiences of my child with special health care needs, his challenges with being bullied, and my attempts to protect him, are similar to many of the stories found in case reports and news articles.

My second child was born in 1990. He was a very quiet baby. I used to call him my "Baby-Baby," because he was so small and fragile. He weighed 5 lb 6 oz at full term, and had to be delivered by emergency C-section because he was in distress. At 9 months old he had tubes put in his ears, when we realized that he could not hear. Once the tubes were inserted, he startled for the first time as he was being driven home from the hospital. How long he had been unable to hear was never determined, but it went back to at least age 6 months and certainly this contributed to delays in his language development.

I worried about his development almost from the moment he was born. Having had a child previously who was typically-developing, I could tell that things were different for this second child of mine. When I asked what was wrong, however, I was told simply that he had developmental delays. At 18 months old, he was referred by the developmental pediatrician for enrollment in an early intervention program. Through the program, he began to receive a range of services including speech and communication therapy, feeding therapy, physical therapy, and special education services. A few years later, he was struggling in his developmental preschool and I requested his medical charts. When I read them, I saw that "autistic like tendencies" were noted throughout the chart, however, the word autism had never been used with me when discussing his condition. Neither I nor his teachers had the advantage of knowing some of the specialized strategies that might be beneficial for his

© Springer International Publishing Switzerland 2015
R. Shetgiri et al., *Practical Strategies for Clinical Management of Bullying*,
SpringerBriefs in Child Health, DOI 10.1007/978-3-319-15476-3_3

development. Those were the days when the diagnosis of autism did not come early. It was when he was almost 6 years old that he received the diagnosis of Autism Spectrum Disorder.

He was a bright and sunny child, except when he was experiencing sensory overwhelm. He seemed very happy in the early intervention environment, even though his language and learning continued to be delayed. When my son communicated in words, he spoke in brief three word sentences. His enunciation was unclear, and only his closest family members and friends could understand what he was saying. Despite this, he experienced great friendship and acceptance from friends and family members. As a young child with a disability, he was well-supported by his small network of family, friends, teachers, and therapists, who knew how to give him the affection, validation, learning, and play opportunities that he needed and wanted.

As the years progressed, it became clear that he thrived in classes that were led by trained autism teachers, and in schools where the principal was actively supportive of children with special health care needs. There was a brief golden age in grades 3–5, where all of the elements were in place for success and acceptance. Not only were the teachers and aides well-trained in autism education techniques, but the school principal was extraordinarily supportive of the children with special health care needs and their teachers. The principal actively modeled interest in, and acceptance of, disabilities and created an environment where students and teachers alike welcomed everyone, regardless of differences. The principal often walked around the school, visiting classes, greeting the children, and interacting with them frequently. It was in this school setting that my son learned the most, interacted with his peers most frequently, and from all outward signs, did not suffer from victimization from bullying. He still had to struggle with the noise that other children made, the scraping of chairs on the floor, the scary sound of the bathroom toilet flushing, the fire alarms, and the commotion in the hallways, but he never came home during those years saying, "Sometimes people mean?"

My son's academic career was a mix of a few great years, some pretty good years, and at least half that were negative, and that put him in the path of bullying. He was victimized by bullying several times over the years, but the victimization became very dramatic during middle school. Middle school is a vulnerable and difficult time for many children, regardless of whether they have disabilities. When my typically-developing older son was in school, parents at his school readily came together several times to act when classmates began to engage in bullying, by organizing mandatory retreats to address the bullying. When my younger son with disabilities experienced bullying at school, however, the school administrators were reluctant to get involved, saying they did not have the time or energy. Connections with other parents in the class did not result in action, because those relationships were more tenuous. The bullying was virtually ignored, even though I sent letters to teachers, principals, and administrators at the district office, and met with the principal and administrators. The difference between the schools my two sons attended was astounding and sobering.

As my child with autism became older, the bullying intensified. He came home from high school saying more and more often, "sometimes people mean?" His informal network of friends and family did not appear to provide as much comfort or support to him as they had previously. This was not because we were not trying, but rather because he was changing. He needed new services and supports that were unavailable or were unsuitable for someone with his sensory issues and particular needs.

In his late teens, after years of such experiences, my son's mental health deteriorated steeply. His descent into anxiety, increased isolation, dangerous behaviors, and aggression, could have been triggered by a number of single incidents, or it could have been a cumulative effect. What was clear was that he felt unsafe and highly stressed, and many of the gains he had achieved when he was younger began to slip away from him. He no longer wanted to go to school, which resulted in missed opportunities for continued education and transition. His mental health issues overwhelmed every other part of his life for several years. I often wonder, how much of this could have been minimized if he had felt safer and happier in his school and community environment?

My son's experience is similar to many other children with special health care needs. Numerous studies have shown that children with special health care needs have higher rates of bully victimization than typically developing children (Twyman et al. 2010). The fallout from bullying is understood more and more to potentially affect the life course. Fortunately, more attention is being focused on bullying and bullying prevention and excellent bullying prevention resources now exist for families of children with special health care needs (See Chapter 6, Resources and Publications). Although they may not have come in time to prevent my son's experiences and subsequent negative outcomes, their existence provides hope and guidance for children and families who are currently dealing with this difficult issue.

Reference

Twyman, K. A., Saylor, C. F., Saia, D., Macias, M. M., Taylor, L. A., & Spratt, E. (2010). Bullying and ostracism experiences in children with special health care needs. *Journal of Developmental and Behavioral Pediatrics, 31*(1), 1–8.

Chapter 4
Bullying and Special Populations

Research findings consistently demonstrate that specific populations are at increased risk of being victimized and/or bullied by their peers, including students with disabilities (Rose and Espelage 2012), sexual minority youth (Espelage et al. 2008), and obese or overweight youth (Adams and Bukowski 2008). Certainly, other youth populations are at-risk (e.g., racial/ethnic minorities, immigrant populations), thus, this is in no way an exhaustive review of those youth that are particularly at risk for victimization or those who are overrepresented as bully perpetrators.

Bullying Among Children with Special Health Care Needs

Children with special health care needs (CSHCN) are defined as those who either have or are at increased risk for having chronic physical, developmental, behavioral, or emotional conditions and who require health and health-related services of a type or amount beyond that generally required by other children (McPherson et al. 1998). CSHCN are at higher risk of bullying and victimization from bullying compared with children without such diagnoses (Twyman et al. 2010). CSHCN also are twice as likely to be bully-victims (Van Cleave and Davis 2006). CSHCN use more care than other children, and are likely to encounter clinicians more often due to their chronic health needs (Van Cleave and Davis 2006). It may be beneficial, therefore, for the clinicians who care for these children, and who are likely to have formed a strong bond with these children and their families, to screen for bullying involvement (Van Cleave and Davis 2006).

Early research on bullying and peer victimization emerged from the field of special education (Hoover and Hazler 1994; Hoover et al. 1993), but a dearth of research addressed bullying experiences among this population until a few years ago. This research indicates that students with disabilities are twice as likely to be identified as perpetrators and victims than students without disabilities (Rose et al. 2011a; Rose and Espelage 2012). In a recent study of bully victimization among students with disabilities using the Special Education Elementary Longitudinal Study and

© Springer International Publishing Switzerland 2015
R. Shetgiri et al., *Practical Strategies for Clinical Management of Bullying*,
SpringerBriefs in Child Health, DOI 10.1007/978-3-319-15476-3_4

the National Longitudinal Transition Study-2 longitudinal datasets revealed a prevalence rate of 24.5 % in elementary school (Blake et al. 2012). Students with disabilities that are characterized or have diagnostic criteria associated with low social skills and low communication skills have a higher likelihood for involvement in bullying incidents (Rose et al. 2011b). Further, a meta-analysis of 152 studies found that eight of 10 children with a learning disability (LD) were peer-rated as rejected; 8 of 10 were rated as deficient in social competence and social problem solving; LD students were less often selected as friends by their peers (Baumeister et al. 2008).

Recent empirical investigations have suggested that victimization may be predicted by the severity of the disability (Rose 2010). For example, students with autism may be victimized more (Bejerot and Mörtberg 2009), and students with learning disabilities may be victimized less than other subgroups of students with disabilities (Wallace et al. 2002; White and Loeber 2008). Studies show that 40–50 % of children who stutter have been teased or bullied about their stuttering, and children who stutter are more likely to be victimized by bullying and to be socially-rejected by peers (Blood et al. 2010). Children with functional limitations or with an emotional, developmental, or behavioral problem are almost twice as likely to be victimized by bullying (Van Cleave and Davis 2006), and children with an emotional, developmental, or behavioral problem are three times more likely to be bullies or bully/victims (Van Cleave and Davis 2006).

To address subgroup differences among students with disabilities, Rose and Espelage (2012) examined rates of bullying involvement and the intersection of individual attributes among middle school students identified with specific disabilities and their peers without disabilities. Students with emotional and behavioral disorders (EBD) engaged in significantly higher levels of bullying and fighting than other subgroups of students. Additionally, higher levels of anger predicted higher levels of bully perpetration for students with EBD, whereas higher levels of victimization predicted higher levels of bully perpetration for students with disabilities other than EBD. These findings demonstrate the importance of recognizing the influence of the characteristic differences between subgroups of students with disabilities, and the unique influence these characteristics may have on student involvement within the bullying dynamic.

Children with attention deficit hyperactivity disorder (ADHD) are almost four times as likely to be victimized by bullying as children without ADHD; relational bullying and ostracism are particularly prevalent in this group (Twyman et al. 2010). Children with ADHD may be victimized due to differences in social development and social interactions (Twyman et al. 2010). Children with cancer, diabetes, and vision problems also are at higher risk of victimization (Van Cleave and Davis 2006).

Autism and Bullying

Children with autism spectrum disorder (ASD) are at particularly high risk for victimization from bullying. ASD consists of a spectrum of neurodevelopmental disorders with prominent features of deficits in social communication and relational problems (Sterzing et al. 2012). Teacher-reported victimization from bullying among adolescents with ASD was 30 %, compared with 17 % self-reported, 7 % peer-reported, and 94 % parent-reported. Bullying perpetration among adolescents with ASD was 46 % by teacher report, 19 % by self-report, and 15 % by peer report (Sterzing et al. 2012). Overall, studies have found that victimization from bullying is higher among adolescents with ASD compared with the general population, whereas perpetration rates are similar (Sterzing et al. 2012). Children who have both ASD and ADHD have increased risk of perpetration (Sterzing et al. 2012; Twyman et al. 2010). Children with ASD experience high rates of relational bullying in the form of social exclusion, with over eight times the likelihood compared with children without an ASD diagnosis; over half of these children experience ostracism (Twyman et al. 2010). Adolescents with ASD who have most of their classes in general education rather than special education settings may experience higher rates of victimization if they are not appropriately integrated into peer groups in general education (Sterzing et al. 2012).

Obesity and Bullying

Weight-based bullying is identified as the most common reason for victimization at 41 %, followed by perceived sexual orientation at 38 %, and intellectual ability or academic performance at school at 10 % (Puhl et al. 2011). It occurs more often than bullying due to race or religion.

Obese adolescents are at high risk of being bullied compared with normal-weight peers (DeSmet et al. 2014; Puhl et al. 2011; Olvera et al. 2013). This weight-based bullying may be particularly damaging in adolescence, an important time for identify formation and peer acceptance. Although it is known that physical appearance, and in particular being overweight, is a major factor in being targeted for peer teasing and ridicule (Hayden-Wade et al. 2005), few studies have examined the subjective teasing experiences of obese youth. One study of perceived stigmatization among overweight adolescent females found that, in this sample of 50 girls, 96 % reported stigmatizing experiences due to their weight, the most frequent occurrences cited as weight-based teasing, jokes, and derogatory names (Neumark-Sztainer et al. 1998). Other studies have found that one-third of adolescent females and one-fourth of adolescent males report victimization from weight-related teasing (Olvera et al. 2013; Puhl et al. 2011); the prevalence of weight-related teasing is 60 % among the most obese students. Obese adolescents also have higher rates of cyber-victimization, with about 12 % reporting cyber victimization in the past 6 months, and are twice as likely to be victimized using electronic media as normal-weight peers (DeSmet et al. 2014). Weight-based victimization of overweight children may begin at an earlier age and last longer than bullying among non-overweight children (Puhl et al. 2013a). Of youth who report weight-based bullying, almost 80 % reported that the bullying lasted for more than 1 year, with more than one in three experiencing it for more than 5 years (Puhl et al. 2013b).

A high proportion of students also report observing weight-based bullying (Puhl et al. 2011). Almost 90 % of students report observing weight-based bullying at school, with less than 5 % stating they have never observed weight-based bullying. Forms of observed weight-based teasing include calling overweight students names, teasing students during physical activity, ignoring or avoiding overweight or obese students, teasing or making fun of overweight students in the cafeteria, excluding them from school social activities, verbal threats, physical harassment, and spreading negative rumors about them. Although the majority of students are willing to help, most report not doing anything when witnessing a peer being teased (Puhl et al. 2011).

In a Canadian sample of over 7,000 youth, Janssen et al. found that overweight and obese children 11–16 years old were at higher risk of victimization from verbal, physical, and relational bullying compared with normal-weight children (Janssen et al. 2004). Boys and girls were equally as likely to be victimized by overt and relational bullying. Obese youth were most likely to be victimized, followed by overweight youth, and the lowest likelihood in normal-weight youth. Overweight and obese boys, however, were no more likely to be physically-victimized than normal-weight boys. Victimization based on weight declined with increasing age among boys, but not among girls.

In this same study, with regard to being a perpetrator of bullying, independent of sex, no associations were detected with BMI status (Janssen et al. 2004). However, associations in bully-perpetrating were found in 15–16-year-old boys and girls; specifically overweight and obese boys were more likely to demonstrate relational bullying compared to their normal-weight peers and associations were also seen for both overweight and obese boys and girls in being more likely to exhibit overt forms of bullying (i.e., name-calling, teasing, hitting, or pushing). Overweight and obese children were more likely to perpetrate verbal bullying by teasing others because of race, color, or religion, but not based on weight (Janssen et al. 2004). It is unclear whether overweight and obese children in this study engaged in perpetration of bullying in retaliation for weight-based victimization.

The likelihood of being bullied may increase by weight status (Brixval et al. 2012; Puhl et al. 2013b). Overweight girls and boys have about one and a half times the likelihood of being victimized, whereas obese girls have more than three and a half times the likelihood (Brixval et al. 2012). The relationship between weight status and bullying may be mediated by body image, with likelihood of victimization increasing with degree of body image dissatisfaction (Brixval et al. 2012).

In a study by Neumark-Sztainer and colleagues (2003), both overweight and underweight middle school students reported higher levels of teasing than average weight participants. Very overweight youth (BMI 95th percentile) were most likely to be teased about their weight; 63 % of overweight girls and 58 % of overweight boys reported teasing by peers, while weight-related teasing by family members was reported by 47 % of these girls and 34 % of these boys. In another study (Hayden-Wade et al. 2005) a significantly higher percentage of overweight students (78 %) reported having been teased or ridiculed about some aspect of their appearance than non-overweight students (37 %). Moreover, the overweight sample was teased significantly more for weight-related aspects of their appearance; 89 % relative to 31.3 %, noting that for the non-overweight children, this percentage included teasing about both underweight and overweight status. Lastly, overweight children reported more frequent teasing, over longer duration, and they found the teasing to be more upsetting, compared with the non-overweight sample.

Weight-based victimization in childhood may predict future overweight (Puhl et al. 2013a). Adams and Bukowski (2008) found that for obese girls, victimization led to higher body mass whereas for obese boys, victimization was linked to decreases in the body mass index. Following preadolescents over 3 years, Lunde et al. (2006) found that early victimization did not predict feelings about appearance, changes in evaluations attributed to others (e.g., how others viewed them), or changes in weight satisfaction. However, for boys and girls being teased about appearance at age ten was linked to more negative self-evaluations and lower weight satisfaction 3 years later.

Overweight and obese children are more likely to experience depressive symptoms compared with normal-weight children (Janssen et al. 2004). Victimization from bullying can further compound this risk. Obese youth who are victimized by traditional bullying are three times as likely to rate lower quality of life, and those victimized by cyber-bullying are five times more likely to have had suicidal ideation (DeSmet et al. 2014).

Weight-related teasing may contribute to negative weight control behaviors, but this relationship may differ by gender. Perceived weight-related teasing is significantly associated with disordered eating behaviors among both overweight and non-overweight boys and girls (Neumark-Sztainer et al. 2003). Degree of teasing also is positively correlated with bulimic behaviors (Hayden-Wade et al. 2005). Neumark-Sztainer et al. (2003) found that weight-body concerns were strongly correlated with unhealthy weight-control behaviors, and family-peer weight norms were correlated with weight-body concerns. After adjusting for family-peer weight norms, however, weight-related teasing was found to be significantly related with weight-body concerns only among boys. Neumark-Sztainer et al. (2003) suggested that girls may be so sensitive to weight norms within their family-peer environments that weight-related teasing does not make any further contribution to weight-body concerns, whereas among boys, the more direct experience of being teased does make an additional contribution. Olvera and colleagues (2013) showed that weight-related teasing is associated with poor body image, binge-eating, and eating disorders among males and females. Teasing from peers and parents was associated with emotional eating, and teasing from parents was associated with binge eating (Olvera et al. 2013).

Overweight and obese children encounter bullying from various sources. Peers are the most common source, followed by parents, siblings, other relatives, and friends (Olvera et al. 2013; Hayden-Wade et al. 2005). Participants in one study reported experiencing bullying by physical education teachers or coaches (42 %), parents (37 %), and other teachers (27 %) (Puhl et al. 2013b). Weight-based bullying from peers and adults may persist even after obese or overweight youth lose weight and have BMIs in the healthy weight range.

Obese adolescents who are bullied demonstrate lower levels of motivation for, and enjoyment of, physical activity (DeSmet et al. 2014). Victims of traditional bullying are more likely to engage in emotional eating and to avoid physical activity and lower-weight peers (DeSmet et al. 2014). Physical education teachers, who may be in a position to intervene in weight-based peer victimization and to encourage physical activity engagement by obese students, may not always intervene appropriately, thereby increasing risk for physical activity avoidance among these students (DeSmet et al. 2014). One study of physical education teachers and coaches showed that participants were more likely to intervene to address bullying of overweight females, but not of overweight males. Female educators were more likely to intervene in bullying than male educators (Peterson et al. 2012).

Youth who experience weight-based victimization prefer intervention by friends, peers, and teachers to cope with the bullying (Puhl et al. 2013a). Less than half of students identify physical education teachers, coaches, or parents as desired agents for intervention. Almost 40 % state that they prefer their parents not to intervene. Adolescents who are victimized more frequently, however, want intervention from all of these groups. Obese adolescents prefer friends and parents to provide support and promote peer inclusion for victims, whereas they prefer that teachers and coaches intervene with bullies to stop the bullying.

It is important to address weight-based bullying and stigmatization in clinical practice with overweight and obese children and adolescents, and in childhood obesity interventions. Obesity intervention efforts and physical activity programs may be more effective if they include components for preventing, identifying, and intervening with weight-based victimization. Studies also show that obese children with higher self-esteem are less likely to be bullied (DeSmet et al. 2014). Obesity intervention programs could incorporate self-esteem management in an effort to reduce victimization. Clinicians can incorporate screening for weight-based victimization in evaluation of overweight and obese adolescents. Providers can also assess children who are bullied for co-morbid mental health conditions and refer them to appropriate mental health services.

Bullying Among Children with Food Allergies

Rates of food allergy are increasing in the United States (Branum and Lukacs 2009), with almost 8 % of children affected by a food allergy (Gupta et al. 2011). Peanut allergy in children has increased from 0.4 % in 1997 to 1.4 % in 2008 (Lieberman et al. 2010). In a survey of parents of children 2–17 years old, 69 % of parents identified allergies as an important health concern for children (Garbutt et al. 2012). Children with food allergies are at risk for being bullied or harassed because of the allergy. In one study of children at an allergy clinic, almost one in four of the respondents reported child victimization due to their food allergy, with the majority of these children victimized more than once (Lieberman et al. 2010). Almost half of children with food allergy seen in a food allergy clinic in New York reported being bullied or harassed; about 1/3 of these children reported being bullied due to their food allergy (Shemesh et al. 2013). Even less frequent events of food allergen related bullying were associated with lower levels of quality of life and higher distress compared with no bullying.

The most common location for bullying due to food allergy was at school, but almost half of respondents stated that the child had been bullied in more than one location (Lieberman et al. 2010). Almost 80 % were bullied by classmates

(Lieberman et al. 2010; Shemesh et al. 2013), and about 20 % of respondents reporting bullying or teasing by a teacher or school staff member. Bullying was done through verbal teasing or taunting, or by having the allergen waved in the allergic child's face (Lieberman et al. 2010). More than half of these bullied children reported being touched by the allergen, having it waved at them, or having it put in their food (Oppenheimer and Bender 2010). Children were bullied by having food waved at them (30 %), being forced to touch the food (12 %), and having food thrown at them (10 %) (Shemesh et al. 2013).

Parents may not be fully aware of their food-allergic children's experiences with bullying. Parents of children with food allergy report lower rates of child victimization from bullying compared to their children's reports (Shemesh et al. 2013). The majority of bullied children (almost 90 %) have reported the bullying to someone; over 70 % told their parents, about 1/3 told a teacher or friend, 20 % told a sibling, and 13 % told a principal. Telling parents appears to help protect children somewhat from the negative mental health consequences of bullying. Children who tell their parents about the bullying report higher quality of life and better social functioning compared with those who have not told their parents (Shemesh et al. 2013).

Bullying Among Lesbian, Gay, Bisexual, Transgender (LGBT) Youth

A large percentage of bullying among students involves the use of homophobic teasing and slurs, called homophobic teasing or victimization (Espelage et al. 2012; Poteat and Espelage 2005; Poteat and Rivers 2010). Bullying and homophobic victimization occur more frequently among LGBT youth in American schools than among students who identify as heterosexual (Espelage et al. 2008; Robinson and Espelage 2011, 2012).

Overall, victimization from sexual orientation and gender expression appears to have decreased in 2011 compared with prior years, however, rates of victimization continue to be high (Kosciw et al. 2012). LGB boys and girls are almost twice as likely to be bullied in high school compared with their heterosexual peers (Robinson et al. 2013). According to the 2011 National School Climate Survey, 82 % of LGBT youth reported being verbally harassed, 38 % were physically harassed, and 55 % were cyber bullied in the past year because of their sexual orientation. Sixty-four percent of youth reported verbal harassment due to their gender expression, and 27 % reported physical harassment (Kosciw et al. 2012). Gender non-conforming students were at particularly high risk of victimization, with almost 60 % reporting verbal harassment due to their gender expression (Kosciw et al. 2012). Eighteen percent of youth were physically assaulted, including being punched, kicked, or injured with a weapon, in the past year because of their sexual orientation, and 12 % because of their gender expression. Transgender students were more likely than other LGBT students to experience victimization, and female non-transgender students were less likely to be victimized and feel unsafe at school. Female respondents reported less victimization related to sexual orientation compared with males and transgender young adults (Russell et al. 2011).

Almost two-thirds of youth reported feeling unsafe because of their sexual orientation and almost half felt unsafe because of their gender expression (Kosciw et al. 2012). Transgender students were most likely to feel unsafe at school, with 80 % reporting that the felt unsafe. Almost 30 % of students skipped class or an entire day of school in the past month because they felt unsafe or uncomfortable. Students who were frequently victimized because of their sexual orientation or gender identity were two to three times as likely to miss school as those experiencing lower levels of victimization, had lower grade point averages, and were less likely to report having plans for continued education after graduation (Kosciw et al. 2012).

The relationship between sexual orientation and suicidality has been shown to be mediated by victimization from bullying (Bontempo and D'Augelli 2002). LGB youth who experience higher levels of victimization are at higher risk for mental health and substance use disorders than their peers. LGB youth who attempt suicide are more likely to report experiencing verbal insults, physical assault, and property damage in the past (Bontempo and D'Augelli 2002). Some LGB youth report greater depression, anxiety, suicidal behaviors, and truancy than their straight-identified peers (Espelage et al. 2008; Robinson and Espelage 2011). Boys who experience bullying due to perceived sexual orientation reported higher psychological distress and more negative views about school than those bullied for other reasons (Russell et al. 2011). Males have higher rates of depression as young adults than females, but this is likely due to higher levels of victimization experienced by males (Russell et al. 2011). Peer victimization in school does not, however, appear to explain all of mental health disparities between LGB and heterosexual youth (Robinson and Espelage 2012), indicating that mental health issues among LGB youth also may be associated with family rejection.

Less than half of LGBT students reported incidents of harassment or assault to school staff due to their belief that the response from staff would be ineffective or would worsen the situation; over one-third of those who did report the incident stated that school staff did not respond (Kosciw et al. 2012). LGB youth living in supportive social environments, which include school anti-bullying policies protecting LGB students, anti-discrimination policies that include sexual orientation, and the presence of gay-straight alliances, are less likely to attempt suicide (Hatzenbuehler 2011). Students in schools with gay-straight alliances report less victimization due to sexual orientation and more intervention from school staff (Kosciw et al. 2012).

References

Adams, R. E., & Bukowski, W. M. (2008). Peer victimization as a predictor of depression and body mass index in obese and non-obese adolescents. *Journal of Child Psychology and Psychiatry, 49*, 858–866.

Baumeister, A. L., Storch, E. A., & Geffken, G. R. (2008). Peer victimization in children with learning disabilities. *Child and Adolescent Social Work Journal, 25*(1), 11–23.

Bejerot, S., & Mörtberg, E. (2009). Do autistic traits play a role in the bullying of obsessive-compulsive disorder and social phobia sufferers? *Psychopathology, 42*(3), 170–176. doi: 10.1159/000207459.

Blake, J. J., Lund, E. M., Zhou, Q., Kwok, O., & Benz, M. R. (2012). National prevalence rates of bully victimization among students with disabilities in the United States. School Psychology Quarterly, 27, 210–222.

Blood, G. W., Boyle, M. P., Blood, I. M., & Nalesnik, G. R. (2010). Bullying in children who stutter: speech-language pathologists' perceptions and intervention strategies. *Journal of Fluency Disorders, 35*, 92–109.

Bontempo, D. E., & D'Augelli, A. R. (2002). Effects of at-school victimization and sexual orientation on lesbian, gay, or bisexual youths' health risk behavior. *Journal of Adolescent Health, 30*, 364–374.

Branum, A. M., & Lukacs, S. L. (2009). Food allergy among children in the United States. *Pediatrics, 124*(6), 1549–1555.

Brixval, C. S., Rayce, S. L. B., Rasmussen, M., Holstein, B. E., & Due, P. (2012). Overweight, body image and bullying – an epidemiological study of 11–15-years olds. *European Journal of Public Health, 22*(1), 126–130.

DeSmet, A., Deforche, B., Hublet, A., Tanghe, A., Stremersch, E., & De Bourdeaudhuij, I. (2014). Traditional and cyberbullying victimization as correlates of psychosocial distress and barriers to a healthy lifestyle among severely obese adolescents – a matched case control study on prevalence and results from a cross-sectional study. *BMC Public Health, 14*, 224.

Espelage, D. L., Aragon, S. R., Birkett, M., & Koenig, B. W. (2008). Homophobic teasing, psychological outcomes, and sexual orientation among high school students: what influences do parents and schools have? *School Psychology Review, 37*, 202–216.

Espelage, D. L., Basile, K. C., & Hamburger, M. E. (2012). Bullying experiences and co-occurring sexual violence perpetration among middle school students: shared and unique risk factors. *Journal of Adolescent Health, 50*, 60–65.

Garbutt, J. M., Leege, E., Sterkel, R., Gentry, S., Wallendorf, M., & Strunk, R. C. (2012). What are parents worried about? Health problems and health concerns for children. *Clinical Pediatrics, 51*(9), 840–847.

Gupta, R. S., Springston, E. E., Warrier, M. R., et al. (2011). The prevalence, severity, and distribution of childhood food allergy in the United States. *Pediatrics, 128*(1), e25–e32.

Hatzenbuehler, M. L. (2011). The social environment and suicide attempts in lesbian, gay, and bisexual youth. *Pediatrics, 127*, 896–903.

Hayden-Wade, H. A., Stein, R. I., Ghaderi, A., Saelens, B. E., Zabinski, M. F., & Wilfley, D. E. (2005). Prevalence, characteristics, and correlates of teasing experiences among overweight children vs. non-overweight peers. *Obesity Research, 13*, 1381–1392.

Hoover, J. H., & Hazler, R. J. (1994). Bullies and victims. *Elementary School Guidance and Counseling, 25*, 212–220.

Hoover, J. H., Oliver, R., & Thomson, K. (1993). Perceived victimization by school bullies: new research and future directions. *Journal of Humanistic Education and Development, 32*, 76–84.

Janssen, I., Craig, W. M., Boyce, W. F., & Pickett, W. (2004). Associations between overweight and obesity with bullying behaviors in school-aged children. *Pediatrics, 113*(5), 1187–1194.

Kosciw, J. G., Greytak, E. A., Bartkiewicz, M. J., Boesen, M. J., & Palmer, N. A. (2012). *The 2011 national school climate survey: the experiences of lesbian, gay, bisexual and transgender youth in our nation's schools.* New York: GLSEN.

Lieberman, J. A., Weiss, C., Furlong, T. J., Sicherer, M., & Sicherer, S. H. (2010). Bullying among pediatric patients with food allergy. *Annals of Allergy, Asthma, and Immunology, 105*, 282–286.

Lunde, C., Frisen, A., & Hwang, C. P. (2006). Is peer victimization related to body esteem in 10-year-old girls and boys? *Body Image, 3*, 25–33. doi:10.1016/j.bodyim.2005.12.001.

McPherson, M., Arango, P., Fox, H., et al. (1998). A new definition of children with special health care needs. *Pediatrics, 102*, 137–140.

Neumark-Sztainer, D., Story, M., & Faibisch, L. (1998). Perceived stigmatization among overweight African-American and Caucasian adolescent girls. Journal of Adolescent Health, 23, 264–270.

Neumark-Sztainer, D., Falkner, N., Story, M., Perry, C., Hannan, P. J., & Mulert, S. (2003). Weight-teasing among adolescents: correlations with weight status and disordered eating behaviors. International Journal of Obesity and Related Metabolic Disorders, 26, 123–131.

Olvera, N., Dempsey, A., Gonzalez, E., & Abrahamson, C. (2013). Weight-related teasing, emotional eating, and weight control behaviors in Hispanic and African American girls. *Eating Behaviors, 14*, 513–517.

Oppenheimer, J., & Bender, B. (2010). The impact of food allergy and bullying. *Annals of Allergy, Asthma, and Immunology, 105*, 410–411.

Peterson, J. L., Puhl, R. M., & Luedicke, J. (2012). An experimental investigation of physical education teachers' and coaches' reactions to weight-based victimization in youth. *Psychology of
Sport and Exercise, 13*, 177–185.

Poteat, V. P., & Espelage, D. L. (2005). Exploring the relation between bullying and homophobic
verbal content: the homophobic content agent target (HCAT) scale. *Violence and Victims*, 20,
513–528. doi: 10.891/vivi.2005.20.5.513.

Poteat, V. P., & Rivers, I. (2010). The use of homophobic language across bullying roles during
adolescence. *Journal of Applied Developmental Psychology*. doi:10.1016/j.aadev.2009.11.005.

Puhl, R. M., Luedicke, J., & Heuer, C. (2011). Weight-based victimization toward overweight
adolescents: observations and reactions of peers. *Journal of School Health, 81*(11), 696–703.

Puhl, R. M., Peterson, J. L., & Luedicke, J. (2013a). Strategies to address weight-based victimization: youths' preferred support interventions from classmates, teachers, and parents. *Journal of
Youth and Adolescence, 42*, 315–327.

Puhl, R. M., Peterson, J. L., & Luedicke, J. (2013b). Weight-based victimization: bullying experiences of weight loss treatment-seeking youth. *Pediatrics, 131*(1), e1–e9.

Robinson, J. P., & Espelage, D. L. (2012). Bullying explains only part of LGBTQ-heterosexual
risk disparities: implications for policy and practice. Educational Researcher, 41(8), 309–319.
doi:10.3102/0013189X12457023.

Robinson, J. P., Espelage, J. P., & Rivers, I. (2013). Developmental trends in peer victimization
and emotional distress in LGB and heterosexual youth. *Pediatrics, 131*(3), 1–8.

Rose, C. A. (2010). Bullying among students with disabilities: impact and implications. In D. L.
Espelage & S. M. Swearer (Eds.), *Bullying in North American Schools: a socio-ecological
perspective on prevention and intervention* (2nd ed., pp. 34–44). Mahwah: Lawrence Erlbaum.

Rose, C. A., & Espelage, D. L. (2012). Risk and protective factors associated with the bullying involvement of students with emotional and behavioral disorders. *Behavioral Disorders, 37*, 133–148.

Rose, C. A., Espelage, D. L., Aragon, S. R., & Elliott, J. (2011a). Bullying and victimization
among students in special education and general education curricula. *Exceptionality Education
International, 21*, 2–14.

Rose, C. A., Monda-Amaya, L. E., & Espelage, D. L. (2011b). Bullying perpetration and victimization in special education: a review of the literature. *Remedial and Special Education, 32*,
114–130.

Robinson, J. P., & Espelage, D. L. (2011). Inequities in educational and psychological outcomes
between LGBTQ and straight students in middle and high school. *Educational Researcher, 40*,
315–330.

Russell, S. T., Ryan, C., Toomey, R. B., Diaz, R. M., & Sanchez, J. (2011). Lesbian, gay, bisexual,
and transgender adolescent school victimization: implications for young adult health and
adjustment. *Journal of School Health, 81*(5), 223–230.

Shemesh, E., Annunziato, R. A., Ambrose, M. A., Ravid, N. L., Mullarkey, C., Rubes, M., et al.
(2013). Child and parental reports of bullying in a consecutive sample of children with food
allergy. *Pediatrics, 131*(1), e10–e17.

Sterzing, P. R., Shattuck, P. T., Narendorf, S. C., Wagner, M., & Cooper, B. P. (2012). Bullying
involvement and autism spectrum disorders. Prevalence and correlates of bullying involvement
among adolescents with an autism spectrum disorder. *Archives of Pediatrics and Adolescent
Medicine, 166*(11), 1058–1064.

Twyman, K. A., Saylor, C. F., Saia, D., Macias, M. M., Taylor, L. A., & Spratt, E. (2010). Bullying
and ostracism experiences in children with special health care needs. *Journal of Developmental
and Behavioral Pediatrics, 31*(1), 1–8.

Van Cleave, J., & Davis, M. M. (2006). Bullying and peer victimization among children with
special health care needs. *Pediatrics, 118*, e1212–e1219.

Wallace, T., Anderson, A. R., Bartholomay, T., & Hupp, S. (2002). An ecobehavioral examination of
high school classrooms that include students with disabilities. *Exceptional Children, 68*, 345–359.

White, N. A., & Loeber, R. (2008). Bullying and special education as predictors of serious
delinquency. *Journal of Research in Crime and Delinquency, 45*, 380–397. doi:10.1177/
0022427808322612.

Chapter 5
School-Based Bullying Prevention Strategies

Most bullying prevention strategies are school-based. Many bullying prevention programs available to schools and communities are not evidence-based. In the past 6 years, however, several meta-analyses have been conducted, and data indicate that the efficacy of school-based bullying prevention programs have varied across countries and contexts (Espelage 2012; Farrington and Ttofi 2011). The most comprehensive meta-analysis that applied the Campbell Systematic Review procedures included a review of 44 rigorous program evaluations and randomized clinical trials (RCTs) (Farrington and Ttofi 2011). Almost 2/3 of the studies were conducted outside of the US or Canada, and 1/3 of the programs were based on the Olweus Bully Prevention Program (Limber et al. 2015). Ttofi and Farrington (2011) found that the programs, on average, were associated with a 20–23 % decrease in perpetration of bullying, and a 17–20 % decrease in victimization (Ttofi and Farrington 2011); however, smaller effect sizes were found for RCT designs in comparison to non-RCT designs. Decreases in bully perpetration included the following program components: parent training/meetings, improved playground supervision, disciplinary methods, classroom management, teacher training, classroom rules, whole-school anti-bullying policy, school conferences, information for parents, and cooperative group work where teachers are taught how to facilitate student group work. Further, the number of elements and the duration and intensity of the program for teachers and children were significantly associated with a decrease in bullying, and the programs worked best with older children (ages 11 and older), and in studies in Norway and Europe in general.

Decreases in *victimization* were associated with the following program elements: disciplinary methods, parent training/meetings, use of videos, and cooperative group work. In addition, the duration and intensity of the program for children and teachers were significantly associated with a decrease in victimization. Work with peers (e.g., peer mentoring, peer mediation) was associated with a decrease in victimization (e.g., Ttofi and Farrington 2011).

Next, three programs that worked best across this meta-analysis are highlighted.

© Springer International Publishing Switzerland 2015
R. Shetgiri et al., *Practical Strategies for Clinical Management of Bullying*,
SpringerBriefs in Child Health, DOI 10.1007/978-3-319-15476-3_5

The Olweus Bully Prevention Program

The Olweus Bully Prevention Program (OBPP) was first implemented in Norway schools, and focuses on reducing existing bullying concerns, preventing new incidents of bullying, and improving school climate and peer relationships (Limber et al. 2015). Program elements focus on restructuring the school environment to minimize the opportunities and rewards for bullying behavior, to shift social norms to create expectations of inclusion and civility, and to build a sense of community among students and adults in the school (Limber et al. 2015). OBPP is based on the need for adults in the school environment to show warmth and positive interests and to be involved with the students, to set firm limits, to consistently use non-hostile negative consequences when rules are broken, and to function as authorities and positive role models (Olweus and Limber 2010). Typically, the components of the program are implemented across the entire school and include specific interventions that are directed at the different level of school's ecology, including hallways, classrooms, individuals, and parents (Olweus and Limber 2010).

There have been many evaluations of the OBPP conducted in many different countries, and the data are limited in the US (Espelage 2013). The studies have produced mixed results, including both positive and negative (null) results, however, it is unclear whether the implementation of the OBPP in all of these studies was consistent with the original OBPP (Olweus and Limber 2010).

The Peaceful Schools Project

The *Peaceful Schools Project,* developed in 2000 (Twemlow et al. 2001) is a philosophy, rather than a program (Twemlow et al. 2004). The Peaceful Schools Project includes five main components. First, schools develop a positive climate campaign that includes counselor-led discussions and the creation of posters that help alter the language and the thinking of everyone in the school (i.e., "back off bullies!" or "stop bullying now"). All stakeholders in the school are flooded with an awareness of the bullying dynamic and bullying is described as a social relationship problem. Second, teachers are taught and coached in classroom management techniques and are taught specific techniques to diffuse disruptive behavior from a relational perspective rather than from a punitive approach. Third, peer and adult mentors are used to help everyone in the school resolve problems without blaming others. These adult mentors are particularly important during times when adult supervision is minimal, such as hallways during passing periods and on the playground. Fourth, the "gentle warrior physical education program" is introduced, and it uses a combination of role-playing, relaxation, and defensive martial arts techniques to help students develop strategies to protect themselves and others. This involves confidence-building exercises that support positive coping. Fifth, 10 min reflection time is included in the school schedule each day. Teachers and students talk at the end of the day about bully, victim, and bystander behaviors. By engaging in this dialogue, language and thinking about bullying behaviors can be subtly altered (Twemlow et al. 2005). In an randomized clinical trial (RCT), elementary students who were assigned to the *Peaceful Schools Project* had higher achievement scores than students from schools without the project; there were also significant reductions in suspensions for acting out behavior in the treatment schools, whereas the comparison schools had a slight increase in suspensions for problem behavior (Fonagy et al. 2009).

KiVa National Anti-bullying Program in Finland

The KiVa program, developed in Finland for elementary through high school students, is a universal school-based program that addresses bullying at school by working with teachers, parents, families, community leaders, and students. Teacher training, student lessons, and virtual learning environments are all critical components of this multi-component program (Salmivalli et al. 2009). Teachers use a manual for classroom instruction, which is supplemented by an anti-bullying computer game for primary school children and an internet forum 'KiVa Street' for secondary school students. On 'KiVa Street', students can access information pertaining to bullying or watch a short film about bullying. Both the anti-bullying computer game and the internet forum are designed to provide opportunities for youth to practice skills learned in the lessons and apply them in different scenarios. Early data show significant decreases in self-reported bullying and self- and peer-reported victimization in 4th–6th graders (Kärnä et al. 2011), and increases in empathy and anti-bullying attitudes.

Social-Emotional Learning Programs

School-based violence prevention programs that facilitate social and emotional learning skills, address interpersonal conflict, and teach emotion management have shown promise in reducing youth violence, bullying, and disruptive behaviors in classrooms (Wilson and Lipsey 2007). This is especially the case for programs that target peer violence in a coordinated fashion across different micro-contexts of the school ecology (e.g., individual, classroom, school, community). Many of these social-emotional and social-cognitive intervention programs target risk and protective factors that have consistently been associated with aggression, bullying, and victimization in cross-sectional and longitudinal studies (Basile et al. 2009; Espelage et al. 2012; Espelage et al. 2003), including anger, empathy, perspective-taking, respect for diversity, attitudes supportive of aggression, coping, intentions to intervene to help others, and communication and problem-solving skills.

Social emotional learning (SEL) programs can be quite diverse in format and intensity, but all have a goal of promoting youth development by building competencies and fostering skills that enable students to flexibly respond to demands and opportunities in their environments (Durlak et al. 2011). SEL approaches focus on students acquiring skills that focus on their ability to recognize and manage emotions, take the perspectives of others, establish and maintain positive relationships and handle interpersonal conflicts appropriately (Elias et al. 1997). More specifically, within the SEL framework there are five interrelated skill areas: self-awareness, social awareness, self-management and organization, responsible problem-solving, and relationship management. Within each area, there are specific competencies supported by research and practice as essential for effective social-emotional functioning, including emotion recognition, stress-management, empathy, problem-solving, or decision-making skills (Elias et al. 1997). Self-regulated learning is both directly and indirectly targeted in these programs. As students are better able to control their feelings, thoughts and actions, especially under emotional demands, academic learning is optimized. Further, exercises and opportunities to practice these skills and competencies differ in their level of cognitive-emotional complexity across development in order to ensure SEL skills are sustainable.

SEL programs use social skill instruction to address behavior, discipline, safety, and academics to help youth become self-aware, manage their emotions, build social skills (empathy, perspective-taking, respect for diversity), friendship skill building, and make positive decisions (Zins et al. 2004). SEL programs offer schools, after-school programs, and youth community centers with a research-based approach to building skills and promoting positive individual and peer attitudes that can contribute to the prevention of bullying.

SEL approaches and programs are quite efficacious in improving academics and decreasing youth violence. A recent meta-analysis including more than 213 SEL-based programs found that if a school implements a quality SEL curriculum, they can expect better student behavior and an 11 percentile increase in academic test scores in comparison to schools with no SEL programming (Durlak et al. 2011). Schools elect to implement these programs because of the gains that schools see in achievement and prosocial behavior. Students exposed to SEL activities feel safer and more connected to school and academics, build work habits in addition to social skills, and youth and teachers build strong relationships (Zins et al. 2004).

Several randomized clinical trials (RCTs) of bullying prevention programs (based on a SEL framework) have attended to the rigorous evaluation of the intervention effects (Brown et al. 2011; Espelage et al. 2013). As schools are increasingly pressed to find time in the day to address psychosocial issues, SEL programs that prevent victimization and its correlates (e.g., social rejection) and also simultaneously improve academic engagement should be rigorously evaluated to make convincing arguments to educators and school administrators that the use of these resources will produce noticeable benefits.

Steps to Respect: A Bullying Prevention Program

Steps to Respect: A Bullying Prevention Program© is designed to help students build supportive relationships with one another (STR; Committee for Children 2001). The Steps to Respect program utilizes a whole-school approach to bullying prevention by addressing factors at the staff, peer group and individual level. Intervening at multiple levels is the most effective way to reduce school bullying, given the complex origins, forms, and maintenance factors associated with bullying. Steps to Respect relies heavily on adults to deliver scripted training from a curriculum and to continually emphasize those lessons throughout the school year.

Empirical support has shown reductions in playground bullying, acceptance of bullying behavior, and argumentative behavior. At the same time, it has demonstrated increases in prosocial student interactions and students' perceived adult responsiveness in comparison with control schools (Frey et al. 2005). More recently, it has demonstrated reductions in physical perpetration, destructive bystander behavior, and increases in bystander behavior and positive social school climate (Brown et al. 2011), especially among schools with high student engagement in the program (Low et al. 2014).

Universal interventions have the potential to reach approximately 80 % of students in a school, which encourages school officials and stakeholders to invest time and effort into these systemic efforts (Walker and Shinn 2002). Thus, the first component of the Steps to Respect program is staff training for "all adults" in the school building, emphasizing that the term includes janitors, bus drivers, mentors, receptionists, school nurses, volunteers, licensed staff, administrators, teachers, assistants, and other adults at school who are involved in the daily lives of students. Training meetings include a scripted training session that provides basic information on the Steps to Respect program, information on bullying, and training on how to receive bullying reports from students. Administrators, teachers, or counselors who will work directly with students who have been bullied or who are bullying others also receive training.

The Steps to Respect curriculum includes lessons to increase students' social – emotional competence and positive social values. Specifically, the program addresses three general skills: First, students learn skills of perspective-taking and empathy and how to manage their emotions. Second, academic skills are also encouraged by incorporating themes of friendship and bullying into literature unit activities such as oral expression, writing composition, and analytical reasoning. Third, the curriculum addresses students' social values by encouraging students' sense of fairness, and attempts to instill a desire for rewarding friendships. Results from Frey and colleagues (2005) demonstrated a 25 % reduction in playground bullying incidents and a decrease in bystanders to bullying episodes who encouraged it compared to a control group. Furthermore, the effects of the Steps to Respect program were most pronounced among students who were observed to do the most bullying before program implementation. Another study reported less observed victimization of all children who had previously been victimized and less destructive bystander behavior among all children who had previously been observed contributing to bullying as bystanders (Hirschstein et al. 2007). In a more recent randomized clinical trial evaluation of Steps to Respect in 33 California schools indicated that participation in a SEL bully prevention program was associated with higher social skills, reductions in aggression, and reductions in bystanders assisting the bully among elementary school children (3rd-6th graders) (Brown et al. 2011).

Second Step: Student Success Through Prevention (Second Step – SSTP)

Second Step: Student Success Through Prevention (Second Step – SSTP; Committee for Children 2008) is the middle school version of the K-8th grade Second Step Program curriculum. Second Step is a social-emotional learning program that also focuses on bullying prevention, sexual harassment, bullying in dating relationships, and substance abuse prevention. The program is composed of 15 lessons at grade 6, and 13 lessons each at grades 7 and 8. Lessons are delivered in one 50-min or two 25-min classroom sessions, taught weekly or semi-weekly throughout the school year. Through skill building and skill practice, the program targets risk and protective factors linked to aggression, violence, and substance use. Curriculum developers also incorporated classic developmental research on risk and protective factors that address simultaneously multiple problems, reducing the need for a separate program for each concern (Hawkins et al. 1999). The program targets the following risk factors: inappropriate classroom behavior, such as aggression and impulsivity, favorable attitudes toward problem behavior (e.g., violence, substance abuse), friends who engage in the problem behavior, early initiation of the problem behavior, peer rewards for antisocial behavior, peer rejection; and the following protective factors: social skills, empathy, school connectedness, and adoption of conventional norms about drug use.

Lessons are scripted and highly interactive, incorporating small group discussions and activities, class discussions, dyadic exercises, whole class instruction and individual work. Delivery of the lessons is structured and supported through an accompanying DVD, which contains rich media content including topic-focused interviews with students and video demonstrations of skills. Manualized training covers not only the curriculum and its delivery, but also an introduction to child developmental stages as related to targeted skills. Lessons are skills-based and students receive cueing, coaching, and suggestions for improvement on their performance. Lessons are supplemented by homework that reinforces the instruction, extension activities, academic integration lessons, and videos. Lessons are supplemented by "transfer of training" events in which the teacher connects the lessons to events of the day, reinforces students for displaying the skills acquired, identifies natural reinforcement when it occurs, and asks students if they used specific skills during the day's events. The program is designed to address directly a range of bullying and violent behaviors including physical, relational and verbal aggression in peer and dating relationships, as well as sexual harassment.

The curriculum targets the peer context for bullying through expanding students' awareness of the full range of bullying behaviors, increasing perspective taking skills and empathy for students who are bullied, educating students on their influence and responsibility as bystanders, and education and practice on the appropriate, positive responses students can use as bystanders to remove peer support for bullying. Students are taught and practice a range of positive bystander behaviors from refusing to provide an audience to directly intervening to stop bullying. By decreasing both active and tacit peer support for bullying, the program is designed to change the peer context, removing the social support that is such a critical driver of bullying and other violent behavior.

Recent research suggests that this program is effective in reducing aggression, homophobic teasing, and sexual harassment. More specifically, an RCT in 36 middle schools found that participants who received SEL instruction via Second Step (Committee for Children 2008) were 42 % less likely to report engaging in physical fights after 6 year in comparison to students in control schools (Espelage et al. 2013) after the 6th grade curriculum (15 weeks). Further, after 2 years of SEL curriculum, students in the Second Step schools were 56 % less likely to report homophobic victimization and 39 % less likely to report sexual violence perpetration than students in the control condition (Espelage et al. 2015). These findings are particularly important given the elevated risk of suicidal ideation and behaviors among youth who are targets of homophobic language, including gender nonconforming and lesbian, gay, and bisexual youth (Espelage et al. 2008; Robinson and Espelage 2011, 2012).

Promoting Alternative Thinking Strategies

The Promoting Alternative Thinking Strategies (PATHS) program, designed for children in kindergarten through sixth grade, was designated a Blueprints model program by the Office of Juvenile Justice and Delinquency Prevention (Kusche and Greenberg 1994). The PATHS program is based on the ABCD (affective, behavioral, cognitive, dynamic) model of development, and places primary importance on the developmental integration of affect and the development of emotion and cognitive understanding as they relate to social and emotional competence (Kelly et al. 2004). The PATHS curriculum builds from a model of development in which children's behavior and internal regulation is a function of their emotional awareness and control, their cognitive abilities and their social skills (Curtis and Norgate 2007). Specifically, the PATHS model posits that during the maturational process, emotional development precedes most forms of cognitive development (Kelly et al. 2004). Following the universal prevention model, PATHS was developed to integrate into existing curricula. Goals of the program include enhancing social and emotional competence and reducing aggression. Some program components are targeted at parents, but classroom teachers, who are initially trained by PATHS project staff, deliver most of the curriculum. The PATHS framework posits that interventions are most effective when the environment promotes opportunities to use the skills that were learned from the curriculum (Curtis and Norgate 2007).

The PATHS curriculum consist of 101 lessons divided into three major units, each containing developmentally sequenced lessons to integrate and build from previous lessons (Curtis and Norgate 2007). The units include readiness and self-control, feelings and relationships, and problem solving (Kelly et al. 2004). There is also an additional supplementary unit that contains 30 lessons. Each unit contains aspects of five themes: self-control, emotional understanding, interpersonal problem-solving skills, positive self-esteem, and improved peer communication/relationships.

Several randomized trials of PATHS have indicated positive outcomes including a reduction in aggressive solutions to problems and increases in prosocial behaviors (Greenberg et al. 2003).

Recognizing, Understanding, Labeling, Expressing, and Regulating (RULER) Approach

RULER is a multiyear program available for kindergarten through grade eight youth, with units that extend across the academic year (Hagelskamp et al. 2013). The design of RULER is based on the achievement model of emotional literacy (Rivers and Brackett 2011) and includes the development of skills to recognize emotions in oneself and others, understand the causes and consequences of emotions, accurately labeling emotions, and express and regulate emotions in an appropriate way (Hagelskamp et al. 2013). Emotional literacy is acquired through the acquisition of emotion-related knowledge and skills; learning skills in safe and supportive environment where the adults model RULER skills; and consistent opportunities to practice using the RULER skills with feedback on their application so that their use becomes refined and automatic. RULER builds social and emotional skills by focusing on the teaching and learning of emotion-related concepts or "feeling words" and by introducing tools for leveraging emotions in the learning environment (Hagelskamp et al. 2013).

The RULER approach includes comprehensive professional development for school leaders and teachers (Hagelskamp et al. 2013). Together, teachers and students analyze the emotional aspects of personal experiences, academic materials, and current events; evaluate how various people, characters, and historical figures feel and manage their feelings; and discuss techniques and use tools for identifying, problem solving about, and regulating their own and others' emotions (Hagelskamp et al. 2013; Rivers and Brackett 2011). Evaluation research shows support for distal outcomes of RULER. Students in classrooms that integrated RULER had greater academic and social achievements compared to students in comparison classrooms

(Brackett et al. 2012). Additionally, longitudinal research has shown that RULER does have sustained impacts on socio-emotional processes in the classroom, and that after prolonged implementation, RULER's impact on classroom quality broadened to include positive effects on the classroom's instructional quality and organization (Hagelskamp et al. 2013).

References

Basile, K. C., Espelage, D. L., Rivers, I., McMahon, P. M., & Simon, T. R. (2009). The theoretical and empirical links between bullying behavior and male sexual violence perpetration. *Aggression and Violent Behavior, 14*(5), 336–347.

Brackett, M. A., Rivers, S. E., Reyes, M. R., & Salovey, P. (2012). Enhancing academic performance and social and emotional competence with the RULER feeling words curriculum. *Learning and Individual Differences, 22,* 218–224. doi:10.1016/j.lindif.2010.10.002

Brown, E. C., Low, S., Smith, B. H., & Haggerty, K. P. (2011). Outcomes from a school-randomized controlled trial of STEPS to RESPECT: a bullying prevention program. *School Psychology Review, 40,* 423–443.

Committee for Children. (2001). *Steps to Respect: A Bullying Prevention Program.* Seattle, WA: Author.

Committee for Children. (2008). *Second step: student success through prevention program.* Seattle: Committee for Children.

Curtis, C., & Norgate, R. (2007). An evaluation of the promoting alternative thinking strategies curriculum at key stage 1. *Educational Psychology in Practice, 23,* 33–44.

Durlak, J. A., Weissberg, R. P., Dymnicki, A. B., Taylor, R. D., & Schellinger, K. B. (2011). The impact of enhancing students' social and emotional learning: a meta-analysis of school-based universal interventions. *Child Development, 82,* 405–432.

Elias, M. J., Gager, P., & Leon, S. (1997). Spreading a warm blanket of prevention over all children: guidelines for selecting substance abuse and related prevention curricula for use in the schools. *Journal of Primary Prevention, 18*(1), 41–69.

Espelage, D. L. (2012). Bullying prevention: a research dialogue with Dorothy Espelage. *Prevention Research, 19*(3), 17–19.

Espelage, D. L. (2013). Why are bully prevention programs failing in U.S. schools? *Journal of Curriculum and Pedagogy, 10,* 121–123.

Espelage, D. L., Low, S., Polanin, J., & Brown, E. (2015). Clinical trial of second step© middle-school program: impact on aggression & victimization. *Journal of Applied Developmental Psychology.* 2015 Jan 2 [Epub ahead of print]. doi:10.1016/j.appdev.2014.11.007

Espelage, D. L., Holt, M. K., & Henkel, R. R. (2003). Examination of peer-group contextual effects on aggression during early adolescence. *Child Development, 74,* 205–220.

Espelage, D. L., Aragon, S. R., & Birkett, M. (2008). Homophobic teasing, psychological outcomes, and sexual orientation among high school students: what influence do parents and schools have? *School Psychology Review, 37,* 202–216.

Espelage, D. L., Basile, K. C., & Hamburger, M. E. (2012). Bullying experiences and co-occurring sexual violence perpetration among middle school students: shared and unique risk factors. *Journal of Adolescent Health, 50,* 60–65.

Espelage, D. L., Low, S., Polanin, J., & Brown, E. (2013). The impact of a middle -school program to reduce aggression, victimization, and sexual violence. *Journal of Adolescent Health, 53*(2) 180–186.

Farrington, D. P., & Ttofi, M. M. (2011). Bullying as a predictor of offending, violence and later life outcomes. *Criminal Behaviour and Mental Health, 21*(2), 90–98.

Fonagy, P., Twemlow, S., Vernberg, E., Mize, J., Dill, E., Little, T., et al. (2009). A cluster randomized controlled trial of a child -focused psychiatric consultation and a school systems- focused intervention to reduce aggression. *Journal of Child Psychology and Psychiatry, 50*(5), 607–616. doi:10.1111/j.1469-7610.2008.02025.x.

Frey, K. S., Hirschstein, M. K., Snell, J. L., Edstrom, L. V., MacKenzie, E. P., & Broderick, C. J. (2005). Reducing playground bullying and supporting beliefs: an experimental trial of the *steps to respect* program. *Developmental Psychology, 41*, 479–491.

Greenberg, M. T., Weissberg, R. P., O'Brien, M. U., et al. (2003). Enhancing school-based prevention and youth development through coordinated social, emotional, and academic learning. *American Psychologist, 58*, 466–474. doi:10.1037/0003-066X.58.6-7.466.

Hagelskamp, C., Brackett, M. A., Rivers, S. E., & Salovey, P. (2013). Improving classroom quality with the RULER approach to social and emotional learning: proximal and distal outcomes. *American Journal of Community Psychology, 51*, 530–543. doi:10.1007/s10464-013-9570-x.

Hawkins, J., Catalano, R. F., Kosterman, R., Abbott, R., & Hill, K. (1999). Preventing adolescent health-risk behaviors by strengthening protection during childhood. *Archives of Pediatrics and Adolescent Medicine, 15*(3), 226–234.

Hirschstein, M. K., Edstrom, L. V. S., Frey, K. S., Snell, J. L., & MacKenzie, E. P. (2007). Walking the talk in bullying prevention: teacher implementation variables related to initial impact of the steps to respect program. *School Psychology Review, 36*, 3–21.

Kärnä, A., Voeten, M., Little, T. D., Poskiparta, E., Kaljonen, A., & Salmivalli, C. (2011). A large-scale evaluation of the KiVa antibullying programme: grades 4–6. *Child Development, 82*, 311–330.

Kelly, B., Longbottom, J., Potts, F., & Williamsom, J. (2004). Applying emotional intelligence: exploring the promoting alterative thinking strategies. *Educational Psychology in Practice, 20*, 221–240.

Kusche, C. A., & Greenberg, M. T. (1994). *The PATHS curriculum*. South Deerfield: Channing-Bete Co.

Limber, S. P., Riese, J., Snyder, M. J., & Olweus, D. (2015). The Olweus bullying prevention program: efforts to address risks associated with suicide and suicide-related behaviors. In P. Goldblum, D. L. Espelage, J. Chu, & B. Bongar (Eds.), *Youth Suicide and Bullying: Challenges and Strategies for Prevention and Intervention*. New York: Oxford University Press.

Low, S., Van Ryzin, M. J., Brown, E. C., Smith, B. H., & Haggerty, K. P. (2014). Engagement matters: lessons from assessing classroom implementation of steps to respect: a bullying prevention program over a one-year period. *Prevention Science, 15*, 165–176.

Olweus, D., & Limber, S. (2010). Olweus bully prevention program. In S. Jimerson, S. Swearer, & D. L. Espelage (Eds.), *International handbook of bullying*. New York: Routledge.

Rivers, S. E., & Brackett, M. A. (2011). Achieving standards in the English language arts (and more) using the RULER approach to social and emotional learning. *Reading and Writing Quarterly, 27*, 75.

Robinson, J. P., & Espelage, D. L. (2011). Inequities in educational and psychological outcomes between LGBTQ and straight students in middle and high school. *Educational Researcher, 40*, 315–330. doi:10.3102/0013189X11422112.

Robinson, J. P., & Espelage, D. L. (2012). Bullying explains only part of LGBTQ-heterosexual risk disparities : implications for policy and practice. *Educational Researcher, 41*(8), 309–319.

Salmivalli, C., Kärnä, A., & Poskiparta, E. (2009). From peer putdowns to peer support: a theoretical model and how it translated into a national anti-bullying program. In S. Jimerson, S. Swearer, & D. Espelage (Eds.), *Handbook of bullying in schools: an international perspective* (pp. 441–454). New York: Guilford.

Twemlow, S. W., Fonagy, P., Sacco, F. C., Gies, M., Evans, R., & Ewbank, R. (2001). Creating a peaceful school learning environment: a controlled study of an elementary school intervention to reduce violence. *American Journal of Psychiatry, 158*, 808–810.

Twemlow, S. W., Fonagy, P., & Sacco, F. (2004). The bystander role of teachers and students in the social architecture of bullying and violence in schools & communities. *Annals of the New York Academy of Sciences, 1036*, 215–232. doi:10.1196/annals.1330.014.

Twemlow, S., Fonagy, P., & Sacco, F. (2005). A developmental approach to mentalizing communities: I the peaceful schools experiment. *Bulletin of the Menninger Clinic, 69*(4), 265–281.

Walker, H. M., & Shinn, M. R. (2002). Structuring school-based interventions to achieve integrated primary, secondary, and tertiary prevention goals for safe and effective schools. In M. R. Shinn, G. Stoner, & H. M. Walker (Eds.), *Interventions for academic and behavior problems: preventive and remedial approaches* (pp. 1–21). Silver Spring: National Association of School Psychologists.

Wilson, S. J., & Lipsey, M. W. (2007). School-based interventions for aggressive and disruptive behavior: update of a meta-analysis. *American Journal of Preventive Medicine, 33*, S130–S143.

Zins, J. E., Weissberg, R. P., Wang, M. C., & Walberg, H. J. (Eds.). (2004). *Building school success through social and emotional learning*. New York: Teachers College Press.

Chapter 6
Anti-bullying Policies and Advocacy

State and National Laws and Policies

There are currently no federal laws directly addressing bullying. Bullying does, however, overlap with discriminatory harassment when it is based on race, national origin, color, sex, age, disability or religion (US Department of Health and Human Services).

State and local lawmakers in many parts of the country have taken action to prevent bullying and protect children. Almost all 50 states have an anti-bullying statute, and most states also have model anti-bullying policies to provide guidance to school districts on how to design their anti-bullying policies (Anti-Bullying Statutes: 50 State Compilation | Network for Public Health Law); (http://www.childrenssafe-tynetwork.org/links/state-laws-bullying-stopbullyinggov). There are significant state and local differences in how these anti-bullying statutes function.

Connecticut, Virginia, New Jersey, Rhode Island, and several other states have particularly well-developed anti-bullying statutes. The New Jersey statute requires each school to appoint an anti-bullying specialist, directs the Department of Education to create a "Bullying Prevention Fund," and institutes state policies to respond to bullying both on and off school property. The Rhode Island Department of Education is directed to create a statewide anti-bullying policy, to provide counseling to victims and bullies, and prohibit students from accessing social networking websites while at school. The model policy for school boards in Virginia addresses bullying through the use of electronics, and recommends that each school board develop a character education program to teach positive character traits and discourage bullying. Connecticut is considered a model state for bullying prevention, with staff routinely receiving calls from other states for guidance on how to build a positive school environment. The Connecticut legislature passed an anti-bullying law which includes mandated training for employees and reporting of bullying incidents. Oregon school districts are encouraged to conduct anti-bullying training sessions and form task forces. In Minnesota, one of the most recent states

© Springer International Publishing Switzerland 2015
R. Shetgiri et al., *Practical Strategies for Clinical Management of Bullying*,
SpringerBriefs in Child Health, DOI 10.1007/978-3-319-15476-3_6

to sign bullying prevention into law, the legislation is considered the result of an essential collaboration between students, educators, administrators, and parents, to help develop safer learning environments for every child in the state.

The United States Department of Education plays an important role in working with the states to ensure that school districts provide safe, nurturing school environments that are conducive to learning. The Office of Special Education and Rehabilitative Services (OSERS) issued a "Dear Colleague" letter in 2013 to provide an overview of a school district's responsibilities under the Individual's with Disabilities Education Act (IDEA) to address bullying of students with disabilities. The letter explicitly states that bullying should not be dismissed, and that school districts need to provide support for students and staff, and create an environment in which bullying does not occur. Bullying of a student with a disability which results in the student not receiving meaningful educational benefit qualifies as a denial of a free appropriate education (FAPE) under the Individual's with Disabilities Education Act. Even when situations do not rise to a level that constitutes a denial of FAPE, bullying can undermine a student's ability to achieve his or her full academic potential.

The work of the United States Department of Education, Office of Civil Rights is equally as important. In the Department's 2010 "Dear Colleague" letter, educators and local school districts were reminded that some student misconduct that falls under a school's anti-bullying policy also may trigger responsibilities under one or more of the federal anti-discrimination laws enforced by the Department's Office for Civil Rights. These laws include protection from discrimination based on race, national origin, gender, or disability, and are enforced by the Office of Civil Rights. The letter encourages educators and school districts to ensure that their bullying and harassment policies comply with these federal mandates.

Best Practices and Advocacy Efforts to Prevent Bullying

The family is undoubtedly the most important place for children to experience empathy and compassion, and to develop emotional wellness, healthy self-esteem, and regard for others. These are vital elements of parenting and child development. Bullying prevention starts, in many ways, with parents learning to incorporate emotional wellness into their own lives and parenting their children with knowledge and confidence. They can be assisted in these efforts through parenting education, and exposure to the American Academy of Pediatrics Bright Futures health promotion themes and recommendations, which are considered the gold standard of pediatric care within the Affordable Care Act.

October: National Bullying Prevention Month

Many agencies and organizations have created promising and best practices to improve outcomes for children who are bullied. A great deal of advocacy revolves around October, which is National Bullying Prevention Month. PACER's National Center for Bullying Prevention created this campaign in 2006, with a one week event which has now evolved into a month-long effort (www.pacer.org).

Advocacy Organizations

PACER's National Center for Bullying Prevention is a leader in developing and providing well-developed strategies and resources to involve partners at all levels, including children, teens, parents, educators, policy makers, and numerous private sector companies and public organizations. PACER educates communities nation-wide to address bullying through creative, relevant and interactive resources, including two interactive websites, KidsAgainstBullying.org and TeensAgainstBullying. org, designed to inspire students to end bullying. PACER's extensive resources are available on line. Their key message is "the end of bullying begins with you." The PACER website contains guidance on how to develop a bullying prevention policy, request a governor's proclamation, influence decision makers, communicate and prepare for a visit with federal and state policy makers, and join in community activities such as Run Walk Roll Against Bullying. They offer bullying prevention and awareness facts, key messages and talking points, current news articles, blogs, and commentary. PACER's National Bullying Prevention Center boasts a large number of private and public partnerships, nonprofits, schools, and community groups who have stepped forward as champions against bullying. These partnerships include organizations such as the National Education Association, American Federation of Teachers, National Association of School Psychologists, Boys & Girls Clubs of America, Gay, Lesbian & Straight Education Network, Girl Scouts of America, The Bully Project, National Association of State Directors of Special Education, and National Autism Society.

Family Voices (www.familyvoices.org) is a helpful resource for families of children with special health care needs and the physicians who work with them. Family Voices is a national organization that aims to provide family-centered care for all children and youth with special health care needs. Family Voices works with the Maternal Child Health Bureau, the American Academy of Pediatrics, and other health quality and health access organizations to connect families of children with special health care needs to best practices and resources for children and youth with special health care needs. Family Voices has State Affiliated Organizations (SAOs) in almost every state, and oversees the work of the federally-funded Family to Family Health Information Centers nationally to ensure access to quality health care and information for families of children and youth with special health care needs and disabilities. Families and providers can access information for the Family to Family Health Information Center in their state, and find out what resources on bullying prevention are available in their area.

The Children's Safety Network (www.childrenssafetynetwork.org) is a National Resource Center for Injury and Violence Prevention, and is dedicated to working with state, territorial, and community Maternal and Child Health and Injury and Violence prevention programs to create an environment where all children and youth are safe and healthy. They work with states and territories to infuse knowledge, expertise, and leadership to reduce injury, hospitalization, disability, and death for all children and youth. Their goal is to equip states to strengthen their capacity, use data, and implement effective strategies to create injury and violence free environments. Bullying prevention is one of The Children's Safety Network areas of focus. They provide data, best practices for prevention efforts, and links to useful publications, webinars, spotlights on various states, and other resources.

The Highmark Foundation (www.highmarkfoundation.org) is a private charitable foundation in Pennsylvania which is dedicated to improving the health, well-being, and quality of life for individuals and communities in their geographic service area. The foundation awards grants to charitable organizations and hospitals that spearhead programs aimed at improving community health. Bullying prevention has been one of their top initiatives for several years, and since 2006 they have been implementing the Olweus Bullying Prevention Program to increase schools' capacities to reduce bullying. Highmark has built a coalition of leaders to work together on bullying prevention, who together were responsible for large-scale implementation of the Olweus Bullying Prevention Program in the United States (Children's Safety Network). The Highmark Olweus project is considered a Promising Practice in Maternal Child Health and brings attention to the dynamics that support a successful partnership. The coalition they developed created a road map for other organizations to use to justify and implement new school-based bullying prevention programs.

"Walk a Mile in Their Shoes" (www.AbilityPath.org) is a valuable collection of stories, resources and data about children and youth with disabilities who face bullying. It describes ways to empower parents and educators to take action and apply meaningful change in the classroom and in the children's lives.

Advocacy Role of Physicians

Physicians can play an enormously important advocacy role, along with principals, educators, parents, and students in promoting knowledge about bullying prevention and sharing resources. Within the clinical setting, physicians can provide families with information about positive discipline, development of their children's emotional wellness, and other aspects of parenting that will assist parents in promoting healthy, empathetic and compassionate children who have healthy self-esteem, and a sense of belonging. Physicians also can act as spokespersons at the community level, adding their voices to bullying prevention activities that local schools and parents are undertaking, and addressing policy makers about the negative impact of bullying on children's health and well-being, and the importance of preventing bullying and victimization.

Role of Public Health in Preventing Bullying

Public health has an important role to play in bullying prevention. The frequent connection of public health nurses and other health care providers with families of young children places them in an important role related to educating about bullying, including how it occurs, signs to look out for, and where to obtain help, support, and resources. Actions that public health departments, healthy communities programs, and others who work in the field can take may include determining what systems and programs are already in place to enforce bullying prevention laws and policies and how the health department is involved in these efforts; helping to coordinate and mobilize partners to support the development of bullying prevention laws and policies; helping to determine which organizations and advocates could serve as effective champions for bullying prevention laws and policies; working with the medical community to include bullying prevention as part of anticipatory guidance; developing and conducting public education campaigns that teach families/parents, community, and children/adolescents about bullying prevention, and their role in prevention; and identifying evidenced based and promising practices and working with internal and external programs to implement them (Children's Safety Network).

An additional area of research that can be further explored is how youth themselves can become part of the bullying prevention research. Youth engagement in participatory research may provide insightful data about bullying prevention, and in the process, exert a positive influence on the youth participants. Participatory research studies with youth demonstrate that this method can help youth develop new knowledge, skills, relationships, and a positive self-identity, qualities that would be beneficial for children and youth involved in bullying.

References

Children's Safety Network Fact Sheet on Preventing Bullying. Available at: www.nihcm.org/images/stories/Bullying_Fact_Sheet_FINAL.pdf. Accessed 11 May 2014.
US Department of Health and Human Services, Health Resources and Services Administration. Available at: www.stopbullying.gov. Accessed 11 May 2014.

Resources and Publications

MCH Knowledge Path on Violence Prevention (www.mchlibrary.info/KnowledgePaths/kp_adolvio.html)
StopBullying.Gov
Teens Against Bullying: A PACER Center website
Kids Against Bullying: A PACER Center website
Bullying: Resource Brief | MCH Library
Special Needs Bullying Prevention Toolkit from PACER and the Bully Project
Walk a Mile in My Shoes, AbilityPath.org
Preventing Bullying in Schools Through Partnerships: a Promising Practices in Maternal and Child Health fact sheet
Social Media and Cyberbullying: Implementation of School-Based Prevention Efforts and Implications for Social Media Approaches
The Cost Benefit of Bullying Prevention: A First-time Look at Savings | Highmark Foundation
Speak Up - Stop Bullying Campaign from Cartoon Network
Teaching Tolerance: Examining Your School's Climate
Preventing Bullying Toolkit from Promote Prevent

Chapter 7
Clinical Management of Bullying

Bullying among children is an important concern for parents. In one study of parents of children 2–17 years old, bullying was one of the top ten health concerns for children and adolescents (Garbutt et al. 2012). Eighty-two percent of parents identified bullying as a health concern for their children; 26 % identified bullying as a "large" problem, 31 % as a "medium" problem. Parents of children 6–11 years old were most likely to identify bullying as a concern compared with parents of younger or older children.

Multiple professional medical societies have issued policies or recommendations regarding bullying and the healthcare provider's role in bullying prevention and intervention. The American Academy of Pediatrics (AAP) issued a policy statement in 2009 entitled "The Role of the Pediatrician in Youth Violence Prevention" (Committee on Injury, Violence, and Poison Prevention 2009). The statement addresses several violence-related issues, including bullying. It is recommended that pediatricians address bullying through clinical practice, advocacy, education, and research. The American Psychological Association issued a resolution on child bullying in 2004 (American Psychological Association 2004). The resolution defines bullying and its consequences and references effective school-based bullying prevention programs. The American Psychological Association resolves to include bullying prevention into its existing violence prevention activities, work with other organizations to disseminate information on bullying, encourage research on bullying and interventions to prevent bullying, and promote the dissemination of culturally-sensitive, evidence-based interventions.

A 2012 Position Statement delineates the role of the school psychologist in bullying prevention and intervention (National Association of School Psychologists 2012). It encourages school psychologists to take a leadership role in developing school-based prevention activities, social skills intervention, evaluate children who bully for social-emotional problems and provide them with pro-social behaviors to implement instead of bullying, counsel victims of bullying, and provide resources and information to parents of children who bully and are victimized about effective strategies and interventions. School psychologists also are encouraged to train

© Springer International Publishing Switzerland 2015
R. Shetgiri et al., *Practical Strategies for Clinical Management of Bullying*,
SpringerBriefs in Child Health, DOI 10.1007/978-3-319-15476-3_7

school staff on bullying interventions, promoting social-emotional development, forming crisis teams, teaching conflict-resolution and social skills, and serve on school crisis and safety teams and monitor the needs of the school regarding aggression and violence.

The American Academy of Child and Adolescent Psychiatry (AACAP) approved a policy entitled "Prevention of Bullying Related Morbidity and Mortality" in 2011 (American Academy of Child and Adolescent Psychiatry 2011). It provides the definition of bullying and its negative consequences. It endorses collaborative efforts by families, healthcare providers, community agencies, and policymakers to prevent and address bullying and its associated morbidity and mortality. The statement says that the AACAP advocates for policy and legislation that promotes awareness about bullying, using evidence-based programs in schools to reduce bullying and increase school safety, encouraging reporting of bullying without threat of retaliation, monitoring and identifying ongoing bullying, accountability for the child who bullies, school-based counseling for victims and perpetrators of bullying, and referrals to healthcare providers to evaluate and address physical and/or psychological symptoms due to bullying. The American Psychiatric Association released a joint position statement with the AACAP endorsing this policy (American Psychiatric Association 2011).

Strategies for Clinicians

There is little information on evidence-based bullying-prevention interventions in the clinical setting. One primary-care-based violence-prevention intervention in the Minneapolis-St. Paul area demonstrated reductions in parent-reported bullying and youth-reported victimization from bullying in the intervention group, compared with the control group (Borowsky et al. 2004). It consisted of mental health screening, referral, and follow-up, and referral to a telephone-based parenting program. The parenting program was adapted from a research-based, parent-training curriculum focused on authoritative parenting and promoting healthy parent–child relationships. The intervention showed larger effects for boys compared with girls.

The AAP Bright Futures guidelines recommend that pediatricians inquire about bullying, beginning with the 5-year-old well-child visit, and continuing through adolescence (Hagan et al. 2008). The recommendations include asking about bullying on the pre-visit questionnaire, discussing bullying if the provider suspects a child is involved in bullying, and providing guidance to children and parents about bullying. Prior studies show that anticipatory guidance about violence prevention is well-received by parents, who believe that pediatricians can help their child avoid violence and can provide education and counseling about community violence (Busey et al. 2006; Barkin et al. 1999). In 2005, the AAP published "Connected Kids: Safe, Strong, and Secure," a primary-care-based youth violence-prevention program (Sege et al. 2005). This program recommends counseling about bullying at the 6- and 8-year-old visits, and provision of a brochure ("Bullying: It's Not OK")

(American Academy of Pediatrics 2006). Program development included focus groups with parents, adolescents, and physicians to elicit opinions on violence prevention topics and to pilot program materials. Parent groups elicited opinions on car safety seats, corporal punishment, and firearm safety, and did not focus on bullying (Sege et al. 2006). Another study using parent focus groups to evaluate the implementation of Connected Kids in a community-based setting examined parental opinions on infancy and early childhood topics (Cowden et al. 2009).

Screening and Identification

Clinicians should ask about bullying at each well-child visit and more frequently for children at high risk for bullying. This could be facilitated by incorporating screening questions into electronic health records or printed pre-visit questionnaires. Bullying should also be in the differential for children who present with psychosomatic complaints, such as headaches, abdominal pain, or enuresis, behavioral problems, mental health problems, and smoking, drug, or alcohol use (Lyznicki et al. 2004). Clinicians can begin simply by asking the child about school and his/her experiences at school. If bullying is suspected, clinicians can probe further to determine the type and extent of bullying, and the child's role in the situation.

Clinicians can educate parents on the negative consequences of bullying for all of the participants, including children who are victimized, children who bully, and those who witness bullying. Parents are often unaware that their children are involved in bullying (Shemesh et al. 2013). Clinicians can teach parents how to recognize signs of victimization such as physical bruises, torn clothes, cuts or scratches, refusal to go to school, worsening academic performance, and nonspecific or psychosomatic complaints such as headaches, abdominal pain, enuresis, sleep difficulties, sadness, or depression (Smokowski and Kopasz 2005; Williams et al. 1996; Schuster and Bogart 2013).

Evaluation and Counseling

Victims of bullying should be evaluated for mental health disorders, such as depression, anxiety, separation disorder, and panic disorder (Lyznicki et al. 2004). Children who bully should be evaluated for conduct disorder and involvement in other high-risk behaviors such as fighting, weapon-carrying, smoking, and drug use (Lyznicki et al. 2004; Shetgiri et al. 2012a). Providers can refer children and parents for further mental health evaluation and intervention (Lyznicki et al. 2004; Shetgiri et al. 2012b). Clinicians can provide parents with information on effective interventions and coping strategies for bullying (Lyznicki et al. 2004). It may be helpful to maintain a list of local community-based programs and treatment resources, accessible to providers and patients thorough electronic health systems or on clinic websites.

Working with Schools

When a child reports to an adult that he/she is being bullied, it is important for that adult to reassure the child that the bullying is not their fault and that they are correct in reporting it to an adult (Lyznicki et al. 2004). If bullying at school is reported to a parent, parents should then discuss the problem with the child's school (Lyznicki et al. 2004). Parents can begin by speaking with the teacher, and if there are no results, the situation can be escalated to the principal or the school board (Shetgiri 2013). Many school districts have procedures for reporting and investigating incidents of bullying. Parents should be encouraged to become familiar with such procedures at their child's school. Parents also can request a change of classroom or seating arrangement for the child, or increased supervision during or between classes. Clinicians can consider obtaining permission from the parents and contacting the school directly about the bullying. Privacy laws may restrict the information that the school can provide about students to those outside their families. As it may be difficult to obtain information on what actions are being taken with the child who is bullying, it is important for parents of children who are victimized to continue to ascertain from the victimized child whether his experience at school is improving.

Strategies for Adults and Child-Serving Organizations

Adults are the role models for children around them. It is important for adults to be aware of their own behaviors, language, and reactions to bullying (Blood et al. 2010). It is important that bullying not be viewed as condoned or acceptable by adults, as this may provide permission for children to bully others. For example, it is important that adults who work with CSHCN treat these children in a way that models respectful treatment by their peers (Blood et al. 2010), and are aware of the indirect messages they may be sending about the acceptability of bullying. Adults need to consistently intervene when children are being bullied. Parents, coaches, teachers, and child-serving organizations who care for overweight and obese children need to be aware of the language used with children, even when encouraging them to lose weight, so that children do not feel blamed or stigmatized for their weight (Schuster and Bogart 2013). Clinicians also should be aware of their language and behaviors when caring for children with stigmatizing characteristics such as obesity, autism, and sexual orientation (Schuster and Bogart 2013). Providers also can pay attention to aggressive behaviors in parents, and help parents modify these behaviors and interactions with their child that may be stigmatizing or bullying (Schuster and Bogart 2013).

Bullying and Social Media

The majority of adolescents access social media sites daily, with more than one out of five adolescents accessing these sites more than ten times a day (O'Keeffe et al. 2011). Cell phones are used by 75 % of adolescents, with more than half using them for texting, and almost ¼ using them for social media and instant messaging (O'Keeffe et al. 2011). Electronic media use is integral to the lives of many adolescents and is the means for communicating with and maintaining their social network. This increase in electronic media use has, however, also contributed to increasing rates of cyber bullying.

Cyber bullying is aggressive behavior using electronic media, with the intent to harm (Kiriakidis and Kavoura 2010). Commonly-used electronic media for cyber bullying include via text messaging or cell phones, Internet websites or chat rooms, email, and computer instant messaging (Kiriakidis et al. 2010). It is more difficult to verify cyber bullying and those who are perpetrating the bullying than in traditional forms of bullying (Kiriakidis et al. 2010; Hinduja and Patchin 2010; David-Ferdon and Hertz 2007). Unlike traditional bullying, which occurs outside the home, cyber bullying follows children into their homes through their computers and cell phones (Agatston et al. 2007). Damaging information posted by bullies on the Internet or communicated via cell phones can reach a wide audience and be disseminated quickly (Kiriakidis et al. 2010; Hinduja and Patchin 2010; David-Ferdon and Hertz 2007). Children who cyber bully do so using various methods. These methods include harassment via threatening messages, spreading rumors, and posting pictures about the victim (Kiriakidis et al. 2010). Sometimes bullies may pretend to be someone else, such as someone the victim knows or admires, to trick the victim to reveal personal information about themselves through email or instant messaging, and then send this information to others (Kiriakidis et al. 2010) or use it against the victim. Bullies also may pretend to be the victim while communicating online and send vicious emails to others or post messages on other children's websites, giving the appearance that they have come from the victim (Kiriakidis et al. 2010). Females are more likely than males to identify cyber bullying as a problem (Agatston et al. 2007). Students are less likely to report victimization from cyber bullying to adults due to fear of losing access to electronic media use (Agatston et al. 2007) and lack of confidence that adults can effectively intervene in cyber bullying (Agatston et al. 2007). Student-used strategies to manage cyber bullying include blocking the sender or the message or ignoring it (Agatston et al. 2007). Requesting removal of websites and posts and helping others who are being cyber bullied were less commonly-used strategies to address online bullying (Agatston et al. 2007).

There are some unique strategies that can be used for cyber bullying. Parents can establish rules about the use of electronic media, including limiting media use time. They can monitor children's Internet use by installing parental controls, bookmarking acceptable websites for younger children, and installing monitoring software when children are older (Kiriakidis et al. 2010). It is important, however, for parents to include these monitoring technologies along with active supervision of their children's online communication, rather than as the sole monitoring method (O'Keeffe et al. 2011). These active strategies could include setting up social networking sites together and knowing their child's passwords, regular checks of children's profiles for inappropriate posts, and parent–child discussions regarding electronic media use (O'Keeffe et al. 2011). Parents also can teach their children about the risks of communication via electronic media and appropriate use of these technologies.

It may be beneficial for parents to improve their own knowledge about electronic media (O'Keeffe et al. 2011). Parents can specifically discuss the potential for easy-accessibility and quick dissemination of potentially destructive information via Internet, email, and text to those besides the intended recipients (Kiriakidis et al. 2010). It is particularly important to talk with children and adolescents about photo-sharing via phone and Internet. Research shows that one out of five teens have shared nude or semi-nude videos or photos of themselves via phone or Internet (O'Keeffe et al. 2011). The Children's Online Privacy Protection Act (COPPA) requires parental permission for websites to collect information on children less than 13 years old (O'Keeffe et al. 2011). Many social networking sites, such as Facebook, have a minimum age of 13 years old to register and have a profile (O'Keeffe et al. 2011). Schools also may have cell phone and Internet use policies and restrictions, and parents should be aware of these school policies (Agatston et al. 2007).

Practical Strategies for Parents

Warning Signs of Victimization from Bullying: Sad, depressed, anxious moods; avoiding school; drop in grades; physical complaints (abdominal pain, headaches, trouble sleeping); torn clothing or bruises

If Your Child Is Being Bullied:

Acknowledge your child's distress

Speak with your child's teacher or school counselor (or adult in charge at the location the bullying is occurring)

Role-play with your child about how to be assertive in possible bullying situations, responding firmly to the bully, with confident body language

Remind your child to stay with friends as much as possible at, to, and from school, especially when there are no adults around

Enroll your child in extracurricular activities that he/she enjoys to help make friends and build self-esteem

Keep a written record of bullying incidents and submit them in writing to the teacher/counselor/adult in charge; document concerns and events in detail (date, description, location, students involved, and whether school staff was aware)

If Bullying Persists

If no response from the teacher or counselor, escalate to principal, school board, or state Department of Education; submit request for intervention in writing

---

Be aware of your state's bullying laws and your child's school's anti-bullying policy

Request class or seat changes if needed

If your child is having depression/anxiety or physical complaints, visit your health care provider. Your child may benefit from mental health services to help with coping skills and assertiveness training

Stop Bullying website: www.stopbullying.gov

National Crime Prevention Council: www.ncpc.org/topics/bullying

Cyber Bullying Website: www.cyberbully411.org

Ophelia Project (parent advice, videos): www.opheliaproject.org/parents.html

Healthy Children Website (Available in Spanish): www.healthychildren. org/english/safety-prevention/at-play/Pages/default.aspx

---

Practical Strategies for Clinicians

Screening
Screen all patients briefly using questions such as, "How are things going at school?", "Do you have friends?", "Is anyone mean to you or picking on you?"

Get a sense of whether they spend lunch/recess with friends or alone

Be cautious about asking children if they are being "bullied" given the stigma associated with the term

If the child seems withdrawn from peers, probe further about teasing, name calling, exclusion

Pay special attention to those with warning signs, special health care needs (e.g. autism, ADHD, obesity, learning disorders), or at high-risk (e.g. LGBT youth)

Always screen children presenting with somatic complaints (e.g. headaches, abdominal pain, sleep problems, bed-wetting)

Initial Management
Acknowledge the child's distress, and reinforce that bullying is not ok, it's not the child's fault

Teach the child to speak calmly to the bully, walk away, and tell a teacher or parent

Encourage parents to practice role-playing with the child to project confidence, and consider enrolling the child in extracurricular activities

Recommend that parents speak with the child's teacher or counselor, document all bullying incidents in detail, and for cyber bullying, print out emails or web posts

If Bullying Persists
Escalate to principal, school board, or state Department of Education

Remind parents to review state and school bullying policy

Recommend that parents request change of classroom or seat, or more supervision during or between classes

Clinicians may be able to help by obtaining parental permission and contacting the school by phone, or by writing a brief letter documenting the concerns

Evaluation and Referral
Evaluate children involved in bullying for depression, anxiety, suicidal ideation, drug or alcohol use, other aggressive behaviors, conduct disorder

Consider referral for mental health services, assertiveness training, coping skills

References

Agatston, P. W., Kowalski, R., & Limber, S. (2007). Students' perspectives on cyber bullying. *Journal of Adolescent Health, 41*, S59–S60.

American Academy of Child and Adolescent Psychiatry Task Force for the Prevention of Bullying. (2011). *Policy statement: prevention of bullying related morbidity and mortality.* Available at: www.aacap.org/aacap/Policy_Statements/2011/Prevention_of_Bullying_Related_Morbidity_and_Mortality.aspx. Accessed 11 May 2014.

American Academy of Pediatrics. (2006). In H. Spivak, R. Sege, E. Flanigan, & V. Licenziato (Eds.), *Connected kids: safe, strong, secure clinical guide.* Elk Grove Village: American Academy of Pediatrics.

American Psychiatric Association. (2011). *Joint AACAP and APA position statement on prevention of bullying-related morbidity and mortality.* Available at: www.psychiatry.org/advocacy--newsroom/position-statements. Accessed 11 May 2014.

American Psychological Association. (2004). *APA resolution on bullying among children and youth.* Available at: www.apa.org/about/policy/bullying.pdf. Accessed 11 May 2014.

Barkin, S., Ryan, G., & Gelberg, L. (1999). What pediatricians can do to further youth violence prevention – a qualitative study. *Injury Prevention, 5*, 53–58.

Blood, G. W., Boyle, M. P., Blood, I. M., & Nalesnik, G. R. (2010). Bullying in children who stutter: speech-language pathologists' perceptions and intervention strategies. *Journal of Fluency Disorders, 35*, 92–109.

Borowsky, I. W., Mozayeny, S., Stuenkel, K., & Ireland, M. (2004). Effects of a primary care-based intervention on violent behavior and injury in children. *Pediatrics, 114*(4), e392–e399.

Busey, S. L., Kinyoun-Webb, C., Martin-McKay, J., & Mao, J. (2006). Perceptions of inner city parents about early behavioral and violence prevention counseling. *Patient Education and Counseling, 64*, 191–196.

Committee on Injury, Violence, and Poison Prevention. (2009). Role of the pediatrician in youth violence prevention. *Pediatrics, 124*(1), 393–402.

Cowden, J. D., Smith, S., Pyle, S., & Dowd, M. D. (2009). Connected kids at head start: taking office-based violence prevention to the community. *Pediatrics, 124*(4), 1094–1099.

David-Ferdon, C., & Hertz, M. F. (2007). Electronic media, violence, and adolescents: an emerging public health problem. *Journal of Adolescent Health, 41*, S1–S5.

Garbutt, J. M., Leege, E., Sterkel, R., Gentry, S., Wallendorf, M., & Strunk, R. C. (2012). What are parents worried about? Health problems and health concerns for children. *Clinical Pediatrics, 51*(9), 840–847.

Hagan, J. F., Shaw, J. S., & Duncan, P. (Eds.). (2008). *Bright futures: guidelines for health supervision of infants, children, and adolescents*. Elk Grove Village: American Academy of Pediatrics.

Hinduja, S., & Patchin, J. W. (2010). Bullying, cyberbullying, and suicide. *Archives of Suicide Research, 14*, 206–221.

Kiriakidis, S. P., & Kavoura, A. (2010). Cyberbullying: a review of the literature on harassment through the Internet and other electronic means. *Family and Community Health, 33*(2), 82–93.

Lyznicki, J. M., McCaffree, M. A., & Robinowitz, C. B. (2004). Childhood bullying: implications for physicians. *American Family Physician, 70*, 1723–1730.

National Association of School Psychologists. (2012). *Bullying prevention and intervention in schools [position statement]*. Bethesda: National Association of School Psychologists.

O'Keeffe, G. S., Clarke-Pearson, K., & Council on Communications and Media. (2011). The impact of social media on children, adolescents, and families. *Pediatrics, 127*(4), 800–804.

Schuster, M. A., & Bogart, L. M. (2013). Did the ugly duckling have PTSD? Bullying, its effects, and the role of pediatricians. *Pediatrics, 131*(1), e288–e291.

Sege, R. D., Flanigan, E., Levin-Goodman, R., Licenziato, V. G., De Vos, E., & Spivak, H. (2005). American Academy of Pediatrics' connected kids program: case study. *American Journal of Preventive Medicine, 29*(5S2), 215–219.

Sege, R. D., Hatmaker-Flanigan, E., De Vos, E., Levin-Goodman, R., & Spivak, H. (2006). Anticipatory guidance and violence prevention: results from family and pediatrician focus groups. *Pediatrics, 117*(2), 455–463.

Shemesh, E., Annunziato, R. A., Ambrose, M. A., Ravid, N. L., Mullarkey, C., Rubes, M., et al. (2013). Child and parental reports of bullying in a consecutive sample of children with food allergy. *Pediatrics, 131*(1), e10–e17.

Shetgiri, R. (2013). Bullying and victimization among children. *Advances in Pediatrics, 60*(1), 33–51.

Shetgiri, R., Lin, H., & Flores, G. (2012a). Identifying children at risk for being bullies in the United States. *Academic Pediatrics, 12*(6), 509–522.

Shetgiri, R., Lin, H., Avila, R. M., & Flores, G. (2012b). Parental characteristics associated with bullying perpetration in US children aged 10 to 17 years. *American Journal of Public Health, 102*(12), 2280–2286.

Smokowski, P. R., & Kopasz, K. H. (2005). Bullying in school: an overview of types, effects, family characteristics, and intervention strategies. *Children and Schools, 37*(2), 101–110.

Williams, K., Chambers, M., Logan, S., et al. (1996). Association of common health symptoms with bullying in primary school children. *British Medical Journal, 313*, 17–19.

Chapter 8
Summation

A large proportion of US children are involved in bullying. Children who bully and those who are victimized by bullying are at-risk for negative short and long-term outcomes including depression, anxiety, and poor psychosocial functioning as adults. Children and adolescents with special health care needs, including learning disabilities, autism, ADHD, and obesity, and LGBT youth are at particularly high risk for victimization from bullying. Evidence-based interventions for bullying are primarily school-based, with whole-school interventions showing the most promising results. Most states in the US now have anti-bullying laws or policies, however, these policies differ by state and locality. Parents, teachers, coaches, and other adults play important roles in preventing and intervening in bullying. Clinicians can prevent and intervene in bullying by screening for and identifying children involved in bullying, evaluating them for co-morbid disorders, referring children and families for counseling, teaching parents how to detect if their child is involved in bullying, how to work effectively with schools, and how to help the child deal with bullying and its consequences. It is essential for everyone who works with children to be educated about the signs of bullying and how to intervene in bullying to prevent its associated negative outcomes.

© Springer International Publishing Switzerland 2015
R. Shetgiri et al., *Practical Strategies for Clinical Management of Bullying*,
SpringerBriefs in Child Health, DOI 10.1007/978-3-319-15476-3_8

Index

© Springer International Publishing Switzerland 2015
R. Shetgiri et al., *Practical Strategies for Clinical Management of Bullying*,
SpringerBriefs in Child Health, DOI 10.1007/978-3-319-15476-3

Printed in the United States
By Bookmasters